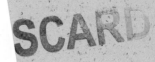

Blackberry Cove Herbal

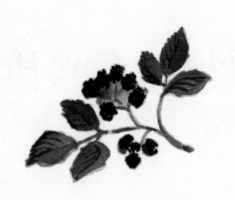

Blackberry Cove Herbal

Healing with Common Herbs
In the Appalachian Wise-Woman Tradition

LINDA OURS RAGO

Capital Books, Inc.
Sterling, Virginia

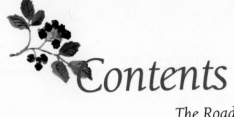

Contents

The Road to Blackberry Cove

Blackberry Cove is an Appalachian mountain farm, a few nearly level clearings tucked up between the rocky ridges. At the foot of its veracious spring it cradles a tiny cabin whose roof was raised by my family and a handful of friends one rainy April in 1973.

My grandfather had bought the abandoned farm in the 1920s to expand his river-bottom holdings nearby and to reclaim the flat spots for orchards of apples and peaches, the sunny spots to grow tomatoes for market. By the time I was a little girl it had once again grown back to tangled blackberry thickets with only a few huge stones still stacked from the hearth of an ancient cabin whose logs had long since molded back into loam. For me it was always a magical place with its crystal water continually pouring from the gnarled roots of a huge sugar maple.

When my children were toddlers we lived in a narrow townhouse convenient to my husband's city job in Washington. On Friday nights we would often bundle everyone up for the long drive from flat tidewater Virginia to our mountains of West Virginia. The rutted lane to the cabin jostled the children awake just long enough to be wide-eyed at the crisp starry sky, undimmed by city lights, before we tumbled them into their beds and lit a warm fire in the stove.

Even before the sun came up over Long Knob we heard the song of spring peepers instead of traffic. There was no telephone, no television, and the children learned water didn't always come out of the spigot. It bubbled up in a sandy pool from the sweet limestone under the mountain.

We eventually moved from lowland Virginia to a more spacious old brick house in the village of Harpers Ferry, West Virginia, where the children grew up. But Blackberry Cove has always been a respite. The walls of our sitting room are covered with photos of the children marveling over salamanders, all of us searching for the first bloodroots and rocking on the porch. Whenever things got hectic or contentious, the cure was usually, "Let's go to Blackberry."

Now the blackberry brambles in the cove have been shaded out by tall hickories and black walnuts. Second-growth sugar maples and white pines grow nearly as tall as the ancient chestnut oaks that have marked the farm boundaries for two hundred years. Fox grapes drape as gracefully as Spanish moss from tree tops, and the forest floor is clear and springy again.

The cabin has settled in as though it had grown like a brown mushroom from under the leaves piled against its walls. The generations of mud daubers on the eaves and the field mice families in the outhouse have become like shirt-tail cousins.

My husband and I and the Shetland sheepdog enjoy peaceful days in the cove, away from busy village life with deadlines, responsibilities, and garden fences. And I have taken to slipping away alone to Blackberry Cove in every season, wandering slowly over her ridges, letting her life unfold around me. At first, I think, it was solace from a house grown quiet after my children moved out to their own lives. Now out of the mountain stillness I feel the low voices of Appalachian grandmothers, and grand-mothers from Scotland and the Black Forest and even older forests. They say, "Listen carefully to the owl." They nudge me to the healing herbs and old books of folklore. They draw me outside when the moon is full and hum lullabies when nights are long.

Their quiet voices have all but been drowned out by shopping malls and cellular phones, but who among us would want to turn back the clock? Even among the fastest moving, though, a small voice often whispers persistently . . . herbal medicine? . . . waxing moon? . . . spring fever?

In the dooryard herb garden at Harpers Ferry the tidy domestic herbs grow contentedly in neat clumps bordered by the old bricks. Their ancestors were nurtured inside the wattled enclosures of village wise women or in the walled gardens of monasteries.

But the Blackberry Cove herbs have always been wild, free to spring up wherever the wind carries their seed. We have watched Mother Nature tend the garden at Blackberry Cove, observing her patterns and wisdom, and trying to walk as gently as we can on her intricate green carpet.

If the herbs are plentiful enough I cut the sprigs I need for "meate or medicine," listening to the grandmothers and silently giving thanks, leaving enough to thrive and propagate. If the herbs are rare or scarce I savor their beauty and form, leaving them to be about their own task of living.

One of the wisest of the grandmothers, Lady Rosalind Northcote, wrote in the early 1900s, "one must feel grateful that the idylls of the forest are still being acted, and that there are still those whose vision is quick enough to catch sight of them and whose pens have the cunning to put before others the glimpses."

This *Blackberry Cove Herbal* is a celebration of the forest idylls, the spiraling seasons, and the animals, herbs, and magic in one small Appalachian mountain cove. May the grandmothers guide my vision and my pen.

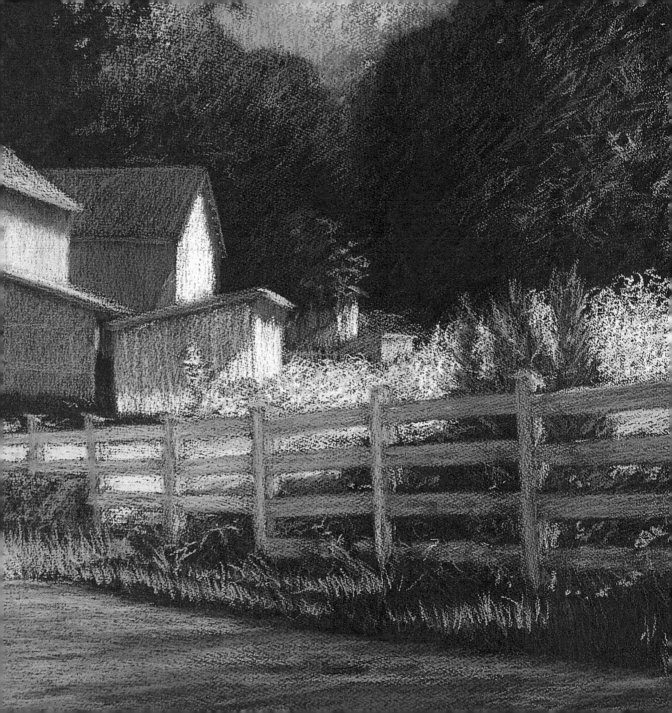

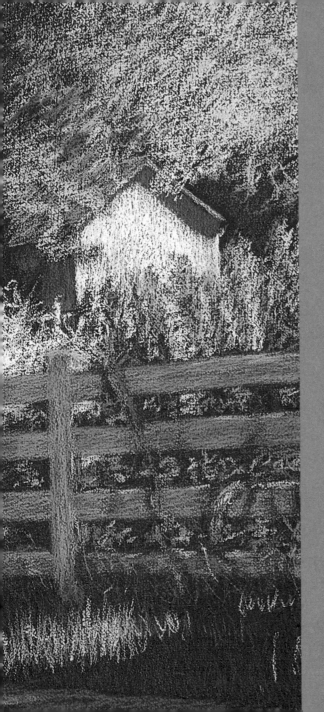

Spring

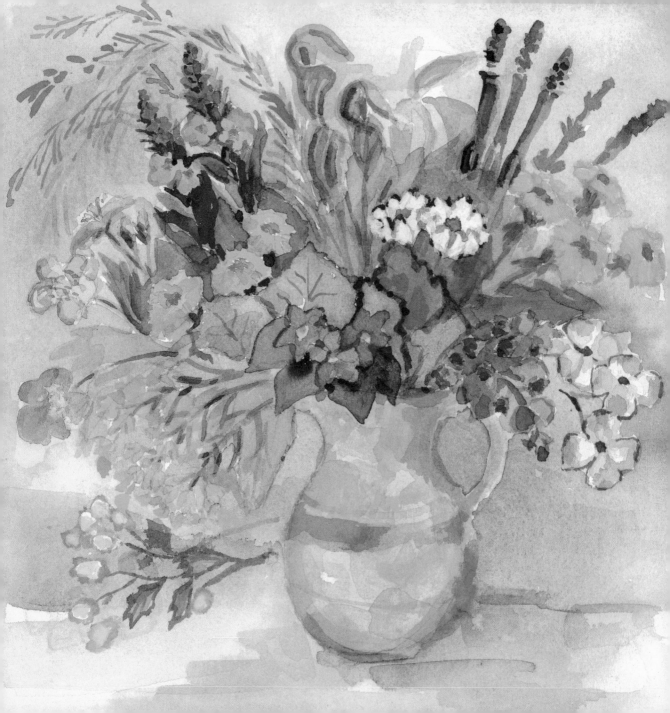

March

The colors of March in Blackberry Cove are still browns and grays, the untidy winter litter. But the second I step out of the car, I smell spring. It is the smell of good clean mud and free water. It is the smell of the sweetness of sap rising in the maples and the first scent of green—not yet chlorophyll, but the whiff of green life nonetheless.

The old willow in the little bog at the end of the lane is nearly quivering with translucent gold. That rising sap will gradually turn the tree to green as the leaves open next month, but for now the luminous amber twigs are the stars of the forest.

And sounds have returned to the cove. At first all I hear is the loud and raucous run, singing its bawdy water song of change back into the land. Then I hear the buzz of a wasp or two already investigating home sites under the eaves of the cabin. Later when I take an afternoon walk to the abandoned homestead in the next cove, I'll hear the hum of the most punctual honeybees — just in time for the first dusting of pollen on bright yellow coltsfoot flowers, the first wildflower to bloom on sunny shale banks. I had driven up to the cabin to look for bloodroots, but it has been a late spring, and it will be nearer the end of March before they send up their striking white flowers with yellow centers.

1. Violet; 2. Yellow Rocket; 3. Black Mustard; 4. Wild Geranium;
5. Coltsfoot; 6. Willow; 7. Mullein; 8. Jack in the Pulpit; 9. Bloodroot;
10. Horsetail; 11. Dandelion; 12. Dogwood; 13. Ground Ivy

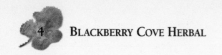

Although the next cove is just over the hill, it is nearly a mile down our lane, out onto the dirt road, and then up Timbrook's winding path to a little cluster of deserted farm buildings. I was enjoying my rest on the sagging corner of the farmhouse porch when a cascade of yellow caught my eye—delicate winter jasmine in its full sunlit glory of blossom. Its surprise brought back images of the old woman, Miss Christina, who had lived there when I was a child. I remember pale flowered cotton dresses on a thin little body and hair pinned up in a wispy gray bun. She swore she had seen a headless man in the gap.

The story was repeated again and again as muggy summer nights settled on my grandmother's wide porch. Miss Christina had come down out of the hills one day to my grandfather's general store. She bought her groceries and then lingered to gossip with the other women on the front steps. When she finally looked up it was later than it had ever been for the walk home. By the time she started back up the narrow track through the deep gap, it was almost dark. Up ahead she saw a man walking slowly, so she hurried a little to catch up and asked if he were walking "clear to the top." He said, "Am." When she turned to look at him, she just had time to see he was headless before he disappeared completely.

I always shivered at that point, no matter how hot the night.

Now I could see her again in my adult mind's eye, sitting here on her sunny step with me, the yellow jasmine flowers uplifting her winter spirit. Where did Miss Christina, in this lonely farmyard, get her exotic winter jasmine? Did my grandmother share a cutting? Grandmother Muriel lived just down the road in an airy valley house surrounded by an iron garden fence filled with colorful flowers and shrubs she ordered from plant catalogues. When I was very little I thought glass canning jars grew in gardens because there were always dozens of them tucked in here and there. I felt so silly when I finally found out they were tiny makeshift greenhouses for rooting sprigs of roses or buddleia.

When the warm sun moved behind the ridge, I stirred from my daydreaming and decided to walk over the top to the upper cove above our cabin. One side of the high little meadow is bordered by remnants of a chestnut rail fence and crumbling stone wall. Did Miss Christina's grandfathers split those rails and lift the stones?

Seep springs had made pocket-sized bogs where the new green grass would be crisp and brown by midsummer. Pale green rosettes of mullein clustered in sunny clearings, their fuzzy leaves warm to my touch. A gray fox resting in the tall grass ahead stood up and watched me for a few seconds before taking off elegantly up the mountain with her bushy charcoal tail barely tipping the rocks.

At that moment it wasn't hard to believe the old tradition that the fox was a fairy spirit who has taken animal form for a little while. Appalachian grandmothers tell that foxes are special friends of the fairies and protect fairy gatherings from mortal intruders. If the fairies are dancing, the fox will lead humans far away.

Witches in these mountains were able to slip out at night and turn into foxes so they could travel secretly and safely. The fox is a "totem" animal, a very powerful magical animal, and tales were whispered around remote cabin hearths about certain families who were actually descended from foxes.

When a sudden shower falls from a clear sky, mountain people say, somewhere a fox is being married. A "fox's wedding" shower is good luck, and you get to make three wishes. One of them will come true! Bury a foxglove flower in moonlight, and the foxes will give you the second sight. Bury one at noon and they will send you gold.

It was good fortune for me to see a single fox, but if I had met several foxes, they would have brought me bad luck.

So I was feeling lucky when I walked the old wood road down into the long purple shadows of our cove where there were still patches of snow under the hemlocks on the northern side. This day had been the essence of spring, but when the sun went down behind the hill, winter returned.

The coals in our stove were banked to last all night, but when startling moon-light awakened me long before dawn, I was glad to have a furry Shetland sheepdog warming my feet.

It was light from the full Worm Moon of March, and I fell back to sleep consider-ing the worms and larvae and seeds and bulbs beginning to loosen the earth in their own ways.

Although it was not yet the Vernal Equinox, I stretched awake early to sunlight–like the March days stretching out daylight on either end, conjuring life back into these ancient hills.

Mullein

Ragged furry mullein (Verbascum thapsus) leaves lie flat on the ground in March, making a perfect pale circle. Smaller leaves cluster upright in the center like cupped green hands around a treasure.

By late June the treasure, a sturdy six-foot staff of mullein flowers, will have risen from that modest wreath. Golden blossoms on the great candelabra will welcome me all along the Blackberry Cove lane. I try to remember some of mullein's folk-names in the English language–king's candle, high taper, candelaria, torchwort, candlewick, hedge taper, Jupiter's staff, Peter's staff, shepherd's club, and Aaron's rod. It's also called blanket leaf, flannel leaf, lady's foxglove, old man's flannel, velvet dock, beggar's blanket, mullkraut, hare's beard, longwort, bullocks lungwort, and Quaker's rouge.

From the length of its distinguished titles, we can begin to understand the honor accorded mullein and how useful it has been to us.

Every variety of mullein is an Old World plant. Our ancestors from Europe must have brought the seeds across the sea in their mattress stuffing, in fodder for their an-imals, or in their pocket lint. I can almost see the hardy seeds sprouting tentatively in the strange New World clearings and then bounding energetically throughout the countryside. Today mullein is a common weed in dry fields and along gravelly road-sides from New England to Missouri and west to the canyons of Arizona. It likes to be center stage, growing best where it is the only large plant.

The tall spikes are actually racemes of blossoms with each corolla consisting of five petals joined only at the base. If you look closely, the lower petals are slightly larger, the one-inch flowers like little cups with tiny seeds inside. Although a single spike will stand until toppled by heavy snows, the flowers along it will open sporadically until late September.

Country people have attributed powerful magic to those tall wands in warding off evil. Dried and dipped in tallow, they were used as torches and lamps.

And the velvety white wool covering the entire plant glows silvery in moonlight. If you look at the mullein hairs with a magnifying glass, you will see each one is branched like a tiny tree, and they grow entangled in a frosty elfin forest.

Seventeenth-century herbalist John Gerard instructs us on how to gather the magical mullein. "Leaves which have not borne flowers gathered when the sun is in Virgo and the moon is in Aries and carried in one's pocket . . . "will prevent fainting, worn by a maiden in her shoe will bring on her menses, and wrapped around fruit will prevent it from rotting.

Our practical grandmothers taught that mullein leaves could be gathered all summer to be used fresh or dried. Tea made with a handful of fresh mullein leaves (half as many dried) in a pint of boiling water, steeped for seven minutes and taken several times a day, is a good cold remedy. Fresh leaves laid on sunburn and other skin inflammations are soothing. Leaves were once dried by Appalachian grannies and smoked in their corncob pipes to ease sore throats and coughs. Mullein leaves were also fed to mountain cattle to cure lung ailments.

Roots are best dug in the fall after the flowers have stopped opening. Boiled in water and mixed with honey or molasses, the root brew is given to croupy children and adults with an "old cough," confided one mountain grandmother.

Mullein flowers are only used fresh. Here is the traditional recipe for an earache remedy. Steep one ounce of macerated flowers in one cup almond oil or olive oil. Let it steep in a warm place (like over a pilot light or on top of the refrigerator) for five days. Apply a few drops in the ear twice a day.

One night an old West Virginia woman with a twinkle in her eye told me how she and her sisters would rub their cheeks with the wooly mullein before their beaus came courting. It gave them a rosy glow!

Whether you use mullein on your cheeks, in your medicine chest, or just to enjoy its stately beauty, honor it and remember how it has been our close companion in life. Let a few plants thrive where they spring up around your house, and they will surely bring you good fortune.

Coltsfoot

Once upon a time nearly every mountain cabin had a box of dried coltsfoot (*Tussilago farfara*) leaves or flowers on the shelf, a ready remedy for winter coughs.

Although its yellow flowers brighten our dry shale banks in March and nearly carpet them with huge green leaves by June, coltsfoot isn't a native to these mountains. Our grandmothers carefully packed up the dried seeds and brought them from the British Isles or northern Europe.

It is easy to understand how the prolific little plant skipped right out of the yarb patch and down the road. I transplanted only one in my small Harpers Ferry herb garden years ago and have rued the day ever since! The pretty dandelion-look-alike flowers soon turn into white puff balls, scattering in the slightest breeze to every corner of the garden. Goldfinches love this white down for lining their nests, and our Scottish great-grandmothers stuffed their pillows with it. At the same time, fleshy little rhizomes are spreading exuberantly underground in all directions.

It is far better to find a sunny hillside along an old wood road for your own coltsfoot patch. In earliest spring it is easy to identify the plant. A scaly stem from two to twenty inches tall, without any leaves, pops up with flowers of numerous rays and a disk. After the flower disappears, large round leaves (sometimes the size of a dinner plate) come up on a long stalk. These leaves are indented on the rim and are smooth but thick, almost leathery. Both sides are covered at first with a soft white down that falls off the top as the leaf expands, but stays on the underside. Before the availability of matches to light fires, this fuzz was sometimes collected for tinder. Coltsfoot's second name, *farfara*, actually comes from Farfarus, or white poplar, to whose leaves it bears a resemblance. Country people thought the leaf looked like a horse's foot, and other folk-names are horsehoof, ass's foot, foalswort, fieldhave, bussfoot, dunhove, hallfoot, and coughwort.

But the botanical name, *Tussilago* (cough dispeller), gives us the clue to coltsfoot's invaluable primary use. In Paris a coltsfoot flower was once painted as a sign on the doors of apothecaries.

Collect the leaves in late June or early July and cut them into strips before drying in a flat pan or basket. They contain mucin, abundant tannin, sitosterol, and zinc. Over the centuries coltsfoot has been used as a demulcent to soothe, relieve, and soften irritated or inflamed mucous membranes. It is not an expectorant that stimulates a cough and expels mucus. This old standby of Appalachian folk medicine gives gentle protective help so healing can take place.

Coltsfoot tea is made by steeping a tablespoon of dried leaves or two tablespoons of fresh leaves in a cup of boiling water for ten minutes. It is traditionally sweetened with honey or molasses.

A mixture of dried coltsfoot flowers, dried mullein flowers, and dried violets is also a traditional cough remedy, made in the same way.

Coltsfoot is also used alone or combined with horehound to make old-fashioned cough drops. Combine coltsfoot and/or horehound tea with two cups of sugar and a pinch of cream of tartar. Cook over low heat until a drop will become hard in a glass of cold water. Pour the mixture in a shallow buttered dish and score into little squares when half hardened. When completely cool, break into pieces and store in a cool dry place.

Our grandmothers were great believers in "herbal tobacco" or the inhalation of burning herbs to cure coughs. This smoking of leaves in pipes seems a little counter-productive today, but coltsfoot flowers were always included in the ingredients.

Willow

Just before the slopes of Blackberry Cove flatten into a small meadow, the run widens out in a spongy marsh. Old Woman Willow tree stood there, huge and grace-ful, for as long as anyone can remember, her roots deep in the moisture, her trunk too thick to encircle with my arms. She toppled several years ago in a violent late win-ter storm, and our whole family mourned.

That summer the great black trunk created a convenient bridge across the swamp for us, as well as other cove creatures, and ground squirrels nested in the dry tangle of her upturned roots.

The next spring a bouquet of vibrant green wands sprang up from that fringe of roots still in water, and now there is a whole grove of new withy-willows!

She is the white willow (*Salix alba L.*). Those silky white branchlets will turn dark when they mature, and the one- to four-inch narrow pointed leaves are glossy green above and white below. The new shoots will someday produce soft inch-long catkin pussies in April and could eventually grow into a seventy-five-foot tree again.

Appalachian grandmothers didn't know willow bark contains salicin, the main ingredient in aspirin, but they knew a tea made from the leaves and bark gathered in late summer would reduce fever and pain. Native American neighbors taught them how to make a strong infusion of bark to treat lumbago and how the catkins sprinkled in soups and stews are an aphrodisiac. Dried willow bark pounded into powder was applied to navels of newborn infants.

Mountain people often call the tree withy or withy-willow and make baskets from the supple stems. Our modern word "wicker" comes from that same source.

The herbalist Gerard wrote in the seventeenth century, "The greene boughs with leaves may very well be brought into chambers and set about the beds of those that be sicke of fevers, for they do mightily coole the heate of the aire, which thing is a wonderfull refreshing to the sicke Patient."

Our ancestors believed plants were whole entities with powers and personalities like our own. We didn't always have to eat or drink them for their cures to work. Just having them about us was sometimes enough.

An old mountain remedy for fever from the German grandmothers is a charm that goes like this: The sick person goes at break of day to an old willow tree and ties three strings around the branches. Then the person says to the willow, "Good morning, old one. I give you my fever. Good morning, old one." Then he or she turns and runs away without looking back.

Here is an old cure for ague (flu or fever). The wise granny asks the sufferer his or her exact name and the precise hour the chill came on. Then the patient is sent to cut the number of withy rods corresponding to that time of day. Thus, if the chill came on at ten o'clock, let him or her cut ten rods. The granny woman then takes the rods and lays them on the fire, saying as each is being put in the fire, "[Name] has the ague. As the rod burns, let the ague burn too." When all the sticks have been burned, the ague will be cured. The patient must look on in silence.

The relater of this charm says, "I know a man who declares that an old woman cured him of most obstinate chills and fevers by this means, but whether every one can do it, I can't say."

April

One April morning we wake up in the cove and it is green. Suddenly! The wave of a magical hazel wand must have passed over the hills while we slept. Of course, millions of small leaves and blades have been uncurling for weeks, but it is on one startling day that their cumulative green changes the whole landscape.

That first green is neon to our winter-weary eyes, and the air crackles with new life. None of us can sit still in April.

A pair of wrens is busy deciding between a perfect nest in a thorny black locust thicket along the lane or one in a crevice around the cabin, and lusty robins are strutting away two by two as they leave the flock and pair off for the season. The dusky brown house wrens (*Troglodytes aedon*) winter over in the cove, clustering together in summer breeding nests for warmth.

The grandmothers know a wren around the house brings good luck, the little bird being domestic but not tamable. She is sometimes called Jenny or Our Lady's Hen and is the bird that makes predictions. Appalachian aunties, rocking on the porch, foretold good fortune or bad by their flight patterns and understood the melodies of wrens. A wren feather found in the wild is the ultimate good luck charm.

This Appalachian reverence for the wren seems to come from Scotland because in England and areas of this country settled by lowlanders, wrens are actually hunted down and killed during the Christmas or midwinter holidays. Some folklorists believe wrens were displaced from high magical status by Christianity. There are many legends and myths about the mighty eagle, representing the pagan sky gods and then later Christianity, battling the tiny earth-goddess wren. She is often portrayed as defeating the larger, more powerful eagle by her wit and cunning. These are always satisfying tales about the humble scoring over the proud.

Here is one of those ancient grandmother stories about the wren.

Once upon a time on a beautiful April morning all the birds decided to choose a ruler. They gathered together in a forest clearing in a huge chattering flock and decided whoever should fly the highest would be their leader. Up they all rose in a great flapping cloud. Soon the small birds were all worn out and fell behind. The big birds flew higher and higher, but none could keep up with the mighty eagle who soared so high he could have poked out the eyes of the sun. When he saw no other bird could fly so high, he turned around and drifted back down to the clearing.

"You are our King," cried all the birds.

"Wait a minute," said the tiny wren, who had hidden in the breast feathers of the eagle. "When the eagle started to come back down, I wasn't tired at all. I slipped quietly out of his feathers and soared even higher. I am your ruler."

And so the wren came to be Queen and ruler of all the birds.

Our beautiful red-breasted robins (*Turdus migratorius*) are often coupled with wrens in our mountain affections. Here are a pair of ditties our great-grandmothers sang to our grandfathers and grandmothers.

Kill a robin or a wren,
Never prosper, boys or men.

The robin and the wren
Are God Almighty's cock and hen.

It is commonly told that whoever kills a robin will have a painful swelling appear on his right hand. If a robin dies in your hand, you will have bad handwriting.

Robins, like wrens, have mysterious powers and a close affinity with us. It is said in the hills that robins can carry fire, and if you kill a robin, your house might burn down.

As prophets of weather, robins singing in high branches always mean fair weather is coming. There is even this little rhyme to make it easier to remember.

If the robin sings in the bush
The weather will be coarse.
If the robin sings on the barn
The weather will be warm.

They appreciate it when we show them our respect, so when a robin finds a dead body in the forest, he will cover the face with moss and leaves to show his respect.

April calls up that ancient urge to clean out the last winter debris, so we give the cabin its annual cleaning. All the windows and door are opened wide, the dusty rugs are shaken clean in the wind, and the last dead wasps who were trapped inside last fall are swept away. Fresh linens get tucked in around the beds, and a crisp new tablecloth with ivy sprigs woven into it is spread on the table. The year is beginning.

I pause for a minute on the porch as a thunderstorm gathers over the head of the cove and watch the magnificence of life-giving and renewing rain, awed at this ritual of resurrection that has been enacted again and again for millions of years.

The first drops hit the tin roof with a din and the wind swirls around in a frenzy, but it's a warm rain without the threat of snow or sleet. The big drops soak into the hillsides to nourish stirring roots and bathe new leaves in encouragement. ·

In West Virginia we call the blue violets Union violets, the white violets Confederate violets, and we're supposed to eat the first violet we see in the spring. When I taste the sweet April violet I give thanks to the whole violet clan for their nourishing vitamin C, for their cheerful beauty, and for keeping their annual promise of springing up in the cove.

The first wood anemones are dangling their delicate white petals, looking deceptively fragile, when in fact they flourish through the last chilly winds and heavy rains of April. Tiny electric blue flowers on the ground ivy are everywhere, and the creamy white dutchman's britches are thick along the shady bank of the gap down to the river. One fat Jack-in-the-pulpit peeks from under his elegant purple canopy.

This year for the first time we have bloodroots appear in our own cove under the paw paws. For many years we took our annual bloodroot pilgrimage to the next cove to admire the exquisite single flower on each plant. I feel because we honored them so, they moved right into our cove with us.

It's hard to leave Blackberry Cove in April. We have an almost uncontrollable desire to witness this vernal urgency, to stand outside and be part of it.

As we reluctantly drive back to Harpers Ferry in the blue evening twilight, we can barely see the newly plowed fields and one farmer still out on his tractor turning over the soil. He must feel it too. Every one of us, animal and plant, is responding to this energy we call spring.

Violets

I gathered a little bouquet of deep purple Union violets and white Confederate violets with butternut gray centers to lay out on the kitchen table at Blackberry Cove. I wanted to identify their particular species in my big *Wild Flowers of the United States* (Rickett). It was a surprise to discover that despite their vastly different colors, they are the same species, *Viola papilionacea*.

The violets are siblings growing on the same hillside, like the boys in this part of West Virginia who also once wore Union blue and Confederate gray. Despite our human hubris, though, we still haven't attained the wisdom of the gentle violet who makes space on the bank for family members of every kind.

Botanists have listed dozens of varieties of violets in nearly every part of the world, but they all hybridize freely. Some plant scholars contend there is no true differentiation—they all form one vast species.

All of them bloom in the spring with that cheerful little pansy face of five unequal petals, the lower one a perfect landing pad for bees. The side petals wear tufts of fine hairs. Five stamens surround five pistils with the lower two stamens exuding nectar that reaches into the spur of the corolla. The fruit is a small capsule that splits into three parts, each bearing a row of seeds.

Curiously, some violet flowers fertilize themselves without ever opening at all, and they also propagate by sending out runners that put down roots. No wonder violets are so common and prolific! In fact, their very name comes from the Latin *vias* or "wayside." Several other flowers were once called "violet," too. Snowdrops were known to our forebears as narcissus violet; lunaria as strange violet; gentian as Marian's violet; and periwinkle as violette des sorciers (the violet of the sorcerers). Our own modern violet was distinguished as the March violet.

As common as they are, we have always loved and used violets. Homer and Virgil relate how Athenians used them to moderate anger, procure sleep, and strengthen the heart. Another old name for violets is heartsease.

The Roman Pliny contended that a garland of violets around the head would dispel the fumes of wine and prevent headaches. Romans even made wine from violet flowers.

A medieval herbal in Britain (Askham's *Herbal*) instructs: "For they that may not sleep for sickness, seeth this herb in water and at evening let him soak well his feet in the water to the ankles. When he goes to bed, bind this herb to his temples."

But some hill folk insist that it is bad luck to bring violet flowers inside because they carry fleas. Our own mountain grandmothers, though, use violets cosmetically. They say that bathing with milk steeped in violets will make a woman irresistible.

And the Appalachian wise women know that violet syrup in equal parts with almond oil is a gentle laxative often given to babies. Here is a recipe for violet syrup:

Violet Syrup

Take a quart of fresh violet flowers. Mash them in a mortar with pestle. Add a quart of water. Mix well and strain. Put the strained liquid over low heat and gradually stir in two cups of sugar. Let it just come to a boil and remove from heat. Bottle and store in the refrigerator.

Violet flowers are rich in vitamin C and contain tiny amounts of salicylic acid. No wonder country children are encouraged to eat the first violet blossom they see in the spring!

The leaves make cooling plasters for inflammations, and the underground roots and rhizomes, dug in the fall, are emetic or purgative.

But the best reason to love and use the little violets is because they are exquisitely beautiful and freely give of their delicate fragrance and flavor. If you are particularly favored you may catch a glimpse of the unicorn stepping lightly among heart-shaped leaves at dawn, cropping violet flowers, her favorite nourishment.

For the rest of us, candied violets may be the closest we get to April enchantment:

Candied Violets

Gather perfect whole violet flowers just after the morning dew has evaporated. Beat an egg white with one-and-one-half teaspoons of water until foamy. Dip each violet blossom into the egg. Sprinkle the dipped violet with granulated sugar until evenly coated. Air dry in a warm dry place. When brittle store them in a tea tin with layers of waxed paper between them. Use within several weeks.

An old cookery book describes a pudding called "Mon amy" that directs the cook to "plant it with flowers of violets and serve it forth."

This is a modern adaptation of another old recipe:

Vyolette

1/2 cup fresh violet petals
1 cup sugar
3 cups water
1-1/2 tablespoons plain gelatin
1 cup orange juice
Whipped cream
Fresh violet leaves

Add violet petals to a boiling syrup of the sugar and water. Simmer covered for twenty minutes. Strain and measure out two cups of syrup. Soften the gelatin in orange juice and add. Pour into individual bowls and chill until firm. Garnish with whipped cream and fresh violet leaves.

Bloodroot

The truest star of our April woodlands is the exquisite white bloodroot flower (*Sanguinaria canadensis*) rising above dry dull leaf litter of last year.

An annual spring ritual in our family is to walk around the mountain and into the next cove where the bloodroots grow in profusion. When the morning sun reaches them on the sides of a deep streambed, some of the flowers are still closed in a creamy white cone while others cup golden stamens in luminous curved petals and still others are wide to the sun in glorious white stars.

Just last spring one or two bloodroots appeared in our own cove. They were drawn, I believe, by our great fondness for them. So I honor them, welcome them heartily, and watch for their numbers to increase.

Bloodroots are perennial natives to North America. They grow on dry open forest slopes in March through May from Quebec to Manitoba and from Florida to Oklahoma. Each flower is like a small magnolia blossom in texture. The heavily veined and deeply lobed leaves only fully unfold after the bloodroot flower has withered. These dark green leaves can become eight inches wide as they cover the seed pod maturing under their canopy.

The leaf and flower stems grow from a horizontal underground rhizome filled with bright red juice, the blood of the root. It is this fat root that is gathered to use fresh by the grandmothers during spring, summer, and early fall.

This root sap was used by Native Americans to dye fabric and as a decorative body stain, as well as medicinally, long before our European grandmothers came to these hills. Puccoon was the Indian name for bloodroot and other dye plants, so the Appalachian settlers called it red puccoon. They also called it Indian paint, tetterwort, red root, coon root, and sweet-slumber.

Only the oldest and wisest grandmothers use the fresh bloodroot sap internally for healing because it can easily become toxic. In dangerous doses it will dim eyesight and cause extreme weakness. Minute amounts were used to ease bronchitis and asthma. It tastes so foul that bloodroot juice was sometimes used to make people vomit up other ingested poisons.

Applied externally, though, bloodroot sap is still an effective home remedy for skin fungus like ringworm or athlete's foot. Until only recently mountain children with eczema (often called "tetter") would show up at school like little woodland Indians, painted with bloodroot.

Ground Ivy

It is only one species of the little European ground ivy (*Glechoma hederacea*) that has made itself so much at home in our hills. Dense little mat by dense little mat, the perennial plant has spread north to Newfoundland and Minnesota and south to Georgia and Kansas. Today there is even naturalized ground ivy along the Pacific Coast.

Hugging the ground are cat-paw-sized dark green leaves with neatly scalloped edges. Square stems only an inch or two tall bear bright purple flowers of inch-long corollas with narrow upper lips and wider three-lobed lower lips.

If you taste a leaf, you will quickly understand why it is considered a bitter herb, but its sharpness is not unpleasant. Our grandmothers have used it like hops to flavor and clarify beer or ale, explaining some of its folk-names of alehoof and tunhoof.

Our family calls it Gill-over-the-ground (Gill or Jill is an old name for a girl or lassie). Others call it Robin-run-in-the-hedge, runaway Jack, Jenny-run-by-the-ground, haymaids, hedgemaids, Lizzy-run-up-the-hedge, and catsfoot.

Gill tea is a cooling old-time drink made this way:

Gill Tea

1 large handful of leaves, stems, and flowers
1 pint boiling water

Steep the Gill-over-the-ground in the hot water for ten minutes. Sweeten with honey. Drink warm or iced.

Mountain grandmothers know Gill tea is a spring tonic. They know it is a good diuretic used for kidney complaints and women with PMS. It is also a home remedy for coughs and congestive headaches. They say the best time to gather the pretty little wild herb to use fresh or dried is in the spring and early summer when it is in bloom.

In fact some grannies ease headaches with a snuff of dried and powdered ground ivy. A generation ago house painters would often use Gill tea to counter the effects of working with lead paint.

So even if you don't actually brew up some Gill tea, next time you notice this diminutive green ally underfoot, give her a nod of respect and recognition.

Jack-in-the-Pulpit

My own mother and grandmother dug up Jack-in-the-pulpit corms (*Arisaema triphyllum*) from shady and damp woodland homes to plant in a place of honor right by the back door. Every spring we would watch for the green spike to push up, the spathe to slowly uncurl, and Jack to arise with all the drama and majesty of an ancient pagan god of the forest.

As a small child I could never reconcile this gentle green Jack with the stern Presbyterian preachers in the pulpit upriver at St. Luke's Church. Only after I had seen the grand canopied pulpits of city churches did I understand the Jack-in-the-pulpit name.

It grows with a large single leaf on a stalk about a foot tall. The spathe forms the pulpit above Jack, which is the top of the spadix. Small inconspicuous flowers are hidden in the base of the spathe, where they mature into a tight bunch of bright red berries by early fall.

The underground corm is called the turnip, inspiring other folk-names of wild turnip, pepper turnip, and Indian turnip. This North American native was eaten after a lengthy cooking process by the woodland Indians. When raw, all parts of the plant are highly toxic, even fatal. There are needle-like crystals of calcium oxalate that cause intense injury to tissue. These crystals are only broken down by cooking for a long time. Other common names are wake robin, dragon root, devil's ear, memory root, dog pint, and cuckoo pint.

Jack-in-the-pulpit is included in this herbal because, like my own foremothers, I revere its strange beauty and the dim memory of its use as nutrition after desperate winters of starvation. And it was once, in long forgotten dosages, the last resort for a beloved child with whooping cough.

Today there is never a reason to ingest Jack-in-the-pulpit! Just enjoy its wonderful presence in the elfin places between our hills.

Dandelion

We all recognize the common dandelion (*Taraxacum officinale*) reflecting the sun itself in spring and early summer. It is an Old World weed from the sunflower family, with hairless and deeply lobed leaves lying nearly flat upon the ground while the glorious yellow flower rays rise from the center.

Who hasn't dispersed the silver plumed seed ball with puffs of breath on a sunny childhood day? The hour of the day and any fortune that can be told with a number are determined by the breaths it takes to blow away every seed. Some folk-names of dandelion are even blew ball, fortune teller, doonhead clock, clock flower, tell time, and puffball. Other descriptive names are lion's tooth, yellow gowns, Irish daisy, and swine snout, while others give us clues to dandelion's heritage in food and medicine: piss-a-bed, bitterwort, cankerwort, and wild endive. Some scholars say the botanical name of *Taraxacum* may come from ancient Greek or Arabic and mean something close to "remedy."

The Appalachian grandmothers never studied Greek, but they know the fresh leaves for salads must always be cut before the dandelion blooms. Roots dug in the spring from two-year-old plants are best for making medicinal teas and cooking in soups and stews. Roots dug in the fall are best for making tinctures, and dried dandelion roots are virtually useless as well as prone to getting maggoty and moldy.

The grandmothers won't tell you that dandelion is rich in calcium, iron, and vitamin A or that it contains vitamin C, potassium, sodium, zinc, and a natural fungicide. But they will tell you that the white "milk" that bubbles up when a dandelion stem is broken will take away warts and heal old sores. They will tell you that dandelion taken in any form is a good remedy for liver and gallbladder ailments and is a gentle diuretic with little stress to the kidneys. Dandelion root tea is a mild laxative.

They will tell you to leave the biggest plant you see because it is the mother plant. Thank her for all the dandelions you gather. And they will tell you the cures work best when you take delight in the dandelion like the bees and little insects who hover over her in the sunlight. Imitate the rabbits who so joyfully eat the dandelion leaves!

Dandelion wine and beer have been favorite country drinks since time began. Here are a few simpler recipes for using the fine healthful dandelion, and don't forget the really easy uses like including unopened buds in omelettes or stir-fries. Make a cup of dandelion tea to soothe a headache by steeping a handful of flowers in a pot of boiling water for ten minutes and sweetening with honey.

Dandelion Broth

1 fat fresh root (per person)
2 cups water (per person)
1 egg (per person)
several fresh sorrel or dandelion leaves

Simmer sliced root for an hour with the leaves. Bring to a rapid boil and stir in the beaten egg. Season to taste, and enjoy right away.

Dandelion Blossom Syrup

1 quart dandelion blossoms
1 quart water
2 pounds of sugar
1/2 lemon

Put blossoms and water in an enamel pot. Bring just to boil. Turn off heat, cover, and let stand overnight. Strain and press the liquid out of the spent flowers. Add sugar and sliced lemon, and heat slowly, stirring now and then, for several hours until reduced to a thick honey-like syrup. Can be kept for several weeks in the refrigerator.

I learned this recipe from Susun Weed who learned the recipe from Maria Treben who learned it from her mother who learned it from a woman she saw carrying a basket of dandelion flowers. I pass it on to you. Who will receive this wise-woman treasure from you? Susun says the days of hand gathering and slow simmering will let you feel the wisdom in this brew.

Dandelion Greens

1 cup fresh dandelion greens (per person)
1/4 cup water (per person)

Wash greens and chop coarsely without drying. Bring water to a boil, add greens, and reduce heat. Cook to your taste–firm or mushy. Add a little vinegar and a dash of salt. Country grandmothers sometimes cooked them with a piece of salt pork and crumbled a hard-boiled egg over them.

Dandelion Aperitif

2 to 3 cups dandelion flowers
2/3 cup of sugar
rind of 1/2 lemon
1 quart vodka

Don't wash the flowers. Cut off the green part. Mix ingredients in a jar and cap. Shake daily. In two weeks strain and enjoy with ice and lemon or in hot water with honey.

Dande-ade

1 quart fresh dandelion blossoms
2 quarts boiling water
3 cups sugar
2 cups cold water
2 oranges, sliced
2 lemons, sliced

Cover blossoms with the boiling water and set aside to cool. Combine sugar with cold water and bring to a boil. Add the sugar syrup, oranges, and lemons to the dandelions and let mixture stand for several days. Strain and serve iced. This can be kept in the refrigerator for a week or so.

May

In May my breath catches at the white magic exploding in the ancient
apple tree standing alone in the little meadow just as I turn into Blackberry Cove.
It is always the first tree I see, welcoming me.

Last February a winter storm cracked it nearly in two, and now a huge gnarled
trunk lies almost on the ground, still hopefully sprouting flowers. In September the
tree gives us knobby sweet apples to nibble between the worm holes. In October it
provides abundant windfalls for the deer, but today there is no mistaking its main
crop—this exquisite loveliness of May. Each white blossom is a perfect tiny rose nestled among pink buds and new leaves no bigger than mouse ears. The tree quivers
with bees, and its fragrance curls up the cove, all the way to the cabin.

When I drive here from Harpers Ferry, over the rolling upland hills in the western
Shenandoah Valley, there are rows upon rows of carefully pruned apple trees blooming in vast orchards. They are a grand sight, but not a wonder. The mystery of apple
blossoms is in one tree we love and know well, all the magic in one ancient branch.

Every tree in Blackberry Cove has darkened now into intense green, and the
shade canopy of the forest is nearly formed. When we stand in the forest in May, we
feel that complex power surging through each tree: moisture and nutrients drawing
up from the earth, charging each leaf with chlorophyll as it transforms sunlight into
energy, nurturing seed and fruit and the roots themselves in unceasing vitality.

That peppery fragrance of May in the cove is pollen so minuscule I can only catch
glimpses of it floating in rays of light or settling like dust on shiny leaves. It is the substance of life from the hickories, walnuts, oaks, and conifers of this Appalachian forest.
Updrafts and breezes through these ridges carry it to the female flowers creating the
seeds that will keep the green of the mountains.

It is a day drizzly with one of those comfortable leisurely rains of May. I am reminded again of how often it rains here, gathering water into rills down the hillsides, making all this green possible, so much moisture that a white mist is lying in the hollows at midday.

The clearing between the cabin and Blackberry Run is thick with field horsetail (*Equisetum arvense*). The thought crosses my mind that someone in the family will have bladder problems this summer. The old-timers said that when an ailment appears, the plant to cure it will often appear too. In any case, this gift of horsetail brushes is as beautiful as any carefully tended lawn.

Although it is still raining lightly, the dog, Tansy, refuses to come inside the cabin. She is deaf and acquiring a cataract along with her arthritis, but she is right. This is no afternoon to be inside. I just push my groceries inside the door, and we take off up the southern slope of Owl Mountain toward the stone wall.

These herbs and wildflowers of May are delicate as they push up from the brittle brown leaves that gently settled last fall on this slope. A medieval tapestry artist could not have imagined a more exquisite field of color than the brilliant, blue-eyed grass (*Sisyrinchium angustifolium*), buttercups (*Ranunculus hispidus*), rue anemones (*Anemonella thalictroides*), and wood anemones (*Anemone quinquefolia*).

I pick my steps carefully to avoid crushing their fragile stems, but Tansy bounds up the hill like a puppy, out of sight over the ridge. While I am climbing over the wall, I see her intensely sniffing something, her small black and white body tense with interest. It turns out to be a pile of fresh horse droppings. Neighbors at the Thompson farm keep horses and are always welcome to ride these old wood roads. There are great clumps of violets along the base of the stone wall, so I think of the author Gladys Taber and how her unicorn came only in May to crop violet leaves along the pond.

Unicorns are horses who have become pure spirit with a burning gold horn on their foreheads to lead them forward on their paths of wisdom. Only the kindest and wisest of our kind can see unicorns.

Horses are a symbol of divine energy and intelligence, and in these mountains a horse is often regarded as the guardian spirit of its owner. It is easy to understand when we consider that until only recently horses plowed the fields that fed us and carried us everywhere, even to our final resting places.

In my own mountain family, the horse evoked an uneasiness. My grandfather was killed long before I was born by a kick to his head from an agitated horse.

Along the run in Blackberry Cove is a wide smooth outcrop of stone where my grandfather's favorite mare slipped and broke her leg. He had to put her down. No other horse ever quite suited, the family always said.

In Appalachian mountain families like ours, a warning called a token is sometimes given just before a death. One night when my father was a boy, the whole family was gathered in the living room as usual after supper. There were my grandfather and grandmother, my father, his two younger sisters, and the schoolmistress, who always boarded with them since the schoolhouse was in sight just across the river. Everyone was quiet. The grown-ups were reading and the children were doing their lessons when all of a sudden they were startled by a loud neighing. "It sounded just like a horse put its head in the window and whinnied," says my father. My grandfather got up and went outside to see if someone was in the yard, but no one was there. The horses were stabled and quiet. "The noise sent shivers down our spines," my father says.

Next morning they heard the news that an old man at the county poor farm across the river had died at just the same time the horse spirit neighed. They all agreed it was a token all right, but I have often wondered if the token might have forewarned of my grandfather's own early tragic death.

So I sit to catch my breath for a minute and ponder this evidence of a horse today. Maybe it was the Celtic goddess Epona, brought over by our great-grandmothers from Scotland alongside their rigid Calvinism. Epona sometimes takes the form of a white horse as she roams these mountains bringing new life. This fertility was remembered and celebrated by our ancestors with their hobby-horses in May Day revels.

The grandmothers say horses are creatures of the moon and their crescent-shaped shoes are especially good luck for women when they are hung up over the door with their "horns" pointing up.

In May bright pink stands of the money plant (*Lunaria*) still bloom in deserted farmhouse yards here. When these blossoms mature into silver moon-like discs later in the season, they have the power to pull the shoes right off any horse's hoof that passes over them in the moonlight.

The grandmothers say horses are able to talk to ghosts and fairies. Witches would try to ride them into infernal realms during the night, so magical plants like mountain ash or stones with holes in them were hung up over the stable doors for protection.

I notice the drizzle stopped while I paused here, so we decide to climb clear to the top of Owl Mountain to try to catch a glimpse of the sun just before it sets. I silently make a wish that no more nightmares find their way into Blackberry Cove, only gentle pleasure horses from over the hill or the white mists of wild benevolent Epona, bringing her May green.

Wild Geranium

A joy of May in Blackberry Cove is the sprawling family of wild geraniums blooming bright purple-rose at the northern base of Owl Mountain.

Those potted red and pink geraniums we carry home from greenhouses are not really geraniums at all but members of the *Pelargonium* genus.

Although there are numerous species of wild geraniums in Europe, this exquisite *Geranium maculatum* is our only native.

Our species has palmately lobed and cleft leaves. The one-inch flowers have five sepals, five petals, and two circles of five stamens—one circle is sterile. Even the pistil is divided into five sections. Five is a magical number to the Appalachian grandmothers, so maybe that is the reason this little geranium is so beloved by them. They say the bluer the flower, the more effective the medicine. The great-great-great-grandmothers from Europe said just having wild geraniums growing nearby could ward off the plague.

When the pistil forms fruit, the mature ovary separates into five parts with a seed inside. Each of these is attached to a part of the long upward-curling style that makes the whole thing look like a long-legged waterbird, a crane.

Cranesbill is another common name for this wild geranium. Other country names are spotted cranesbill, wild cranesbill, storksbill, sweet Indian storksbill, alum root, alum bloom, chocolate flower, crowfoot, dove's-foot, old maid's nightcap, shameface, and pinchneedle.

It is the dried or fresh leaves and the dried or fresh fat underground rhizome that is used as a bitter tea to restore lost strength or settle windiness in the gut. Other traditional uses for the tea are to apply it externally to ease piles or as a gargle for sore throats.

To get the best effect medicinally, the root or rhizome should be dug near the dark of the moon in the cycle just before the plant blooms. The leaves should be gathered at the full moon before the plant blooms. Either can be used fresh or dried.

Here is the method for making cranesbill tea or infusion:

<u>*Wild Geranium Tea*</u>

1 ounce dried plant material
or
2 ounces fresh plant material
1 pint boiling water

Pour the boiling water over cranesbill and steep for ten minutes. Use right away after it cools a little. When taken internally, sweeten the tea with honey.

Horsetail

A tiny sloping meadow falls gradually from the cabin's front door to Blackberry Run. Last spring it was alive with a whole herd of bright green horsetail (*Equisetum arvense*), as if the bright plumes had galloped in for the first time during the night.

These beautiful eight- to ten-inch stalks of horsetail are ancient plants, closely related to ferns, and, like ferns, they were as big as trees during the dinosaur age. They love growing in places where their perennial underground rhizomes can pull up moisture from underground streams, so country water dowsers keep an eye out for horsetails.

The plant has no leaves, just its distinctive jointed bristles that rise directly from the ground and contain valuable silica. The great-grandmothers used horsetails to scour pewter chargers, and the grandmothers used them to make milk pans shine. Some folk-names are shave grass, bottle brush, paddock pipes, Dutch rushes (lots of pewter was made in Holland), and pewterwort.

The fertile stems of horsetail bear a cone-like catkin of spores, but these wither quickly. It is the hardy infertile ones we use. Cut them off right at the ground and use fresh or hang up to dry in a dark dry place with good ventilation.

Dried horsetail is traditionally tied up in a handkerchief and steeped in a hot bath to relieve aches and pains of rheumatism, sore muscles, or arthritis.

Ashes of dried horsetails are the country remedy for too much stomach acid. A few grains of the ashes in a cup of tea is the usual prescription.

Horsetail is astringent, so it is used both dried and fresh to help stop light external bleeding. A favorite mountain way to stop a nosebleed is to sniffle up the following decoction. Bladder infection, though, is the most common ailment for which our grandmothers prescribed this remedy.

Horsetail Decoction

1 cup of boiling water poured on
1 teaspoon dried horsetail or
2 teaspoons fresh horsetail

Infuse for twenty minutes. Take this three times a day.

Horsetail is best used in small frequent doses. Do not use for more than a month as it can irritate the kidneys.

Mustard

Our wild black mustard (*Brassica kaber*) blooms in brilliant yellow flowers on scraggly waste areas from May to July. The clump I harvest from at Blackberry Cove is tucked up on a shaly bank across from our lane. It has naturalized from a farmhouse garden, so I like to think the cheerful upright plants are descendants of the mustard around Blackberry Cove's original log cabin nearly two hundred years ago.

The women who gardened there may have called it sinap or winter cress. They knew chewing the fresh leaves eases a toothache or seeds steeped in vinegar are a remedy for upset stomachs or a poor appetite.

The grandmothers knew mustard applied externally is a rubefacient—it stimulates blood flow to help in healing. Here is the traditional method:

Mustard Plaster

1 tablespoon powdered mustard seed (purchased or homemade)
1 quart cold water

Combine and stir over heat until the water is comfortably warm to the touch. Saturate a towel in the mustard water, wring it out, and lay it across the chest for coughs. Lay the towel on other areas with infections also.

This mustard water also makes a good footbath to ease headaches.

Do not leave a mustard water towel on for more than ten minutes at a time because it can cause the skin to blister.

Today we are more inclined to buy our mustard in a jar, already prepared with vinegar and spices. The grannies knew the taste of mustard "quickens and revives the spirit." We still like it to add flavor and an attractive pungency to cold meats and sandwiches. One very wise mountain woman told me, "If you don't relish your dinner, you won't digest it right."

Yellow Rocket

I have included this close relative of mustard (*Barbarea vulgaris*) because it is so often mistaken for wild mustard. This yellow rocket is also called winter cress and can cover a whole field in these hills in late spring. It is easy to distinguish from the true mustards if you look closely at the stems. The mustard stem is bristly or hairy, and the yellow rocket stem is smooth. Mustard flowers turn into a long pod with an angled beak containing the familiar round mustard seeds.

This yellow rocket is good in its own right as a salad herb. Its leaves are strong-tasting, but add a wonderful bite to lettuce and purslane. For salads the leaves should be gathered before flowering.

To use yellow rocket for medicine, you should gather the leaves after flowering. The grandmothers teach that the seeds "stir up bodily lust and provoke urine." The roots steeped in vinegar and applied externally are said to take away freckles!

Dogwood

This year it is the first week of May when white starbursts explode like Fourth of July fireworks on the ridges around Blackberry Cove. Up close I can see each one is a little dogwood (*Cornus florida*), our exquisite native tree.

Some stand sparkling white in the newly greening forest, and others tangle into pink hazy drifts of blooming redbuds to create whole groves of wild May Day enchantment.

Dogwood trees love the rich shady forest understory on the slopes of these eastern Appalachian foothills, but even in these ideal conditions they rarely grow taller than fifteen feet. By fall each stemless white flower with its four petals will gradually mature into a dense cluster of red berries, lasting all winter until the birds have eaten every one.

The grandmothers' winter-weary spirits were uplifted by the dogwood too, and it reminded them to harvest and dry the flowers, root bark, and inner bark from now at blooming time until first frost.

The root bark can be boiled in water to make a rub for aching muscles. Grandmothers boiled the inner bark in water to treat "loose bowels."

Before the days of commercial toothpaste, mountain people pounded the dried inner bark into a cleansing and healing tooth powder. I cut a twig to try the old way of making a toothbrush by fraying the end into a little bristle. It has a sweet and delicate taste, and for about a week it works nearly as well as my store-bought one of plastic.

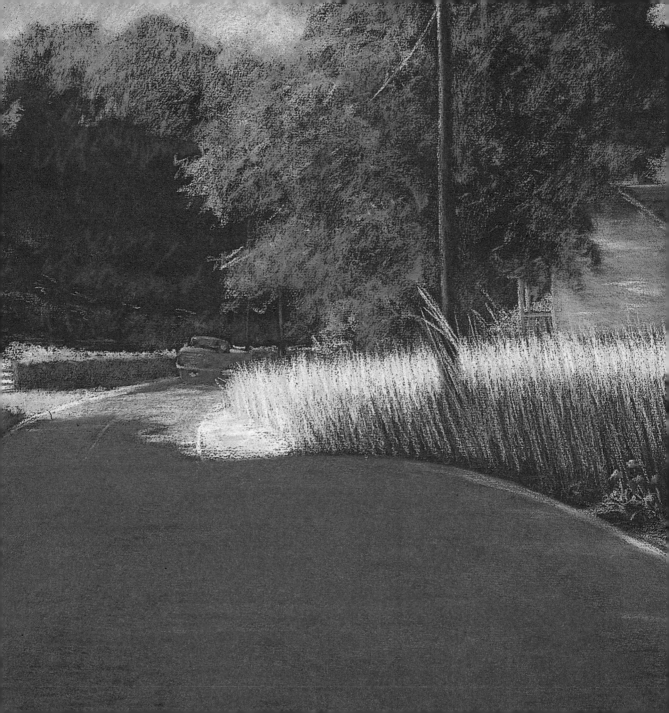

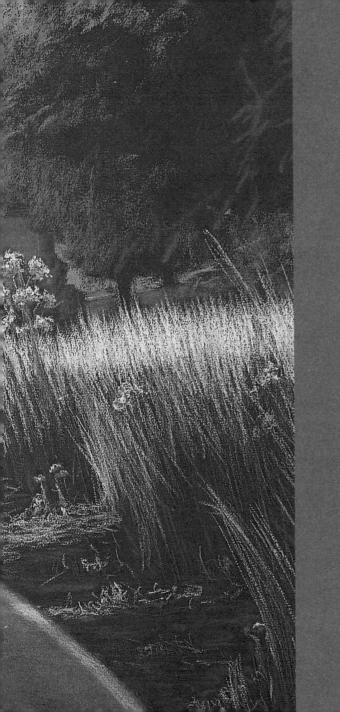

Summer

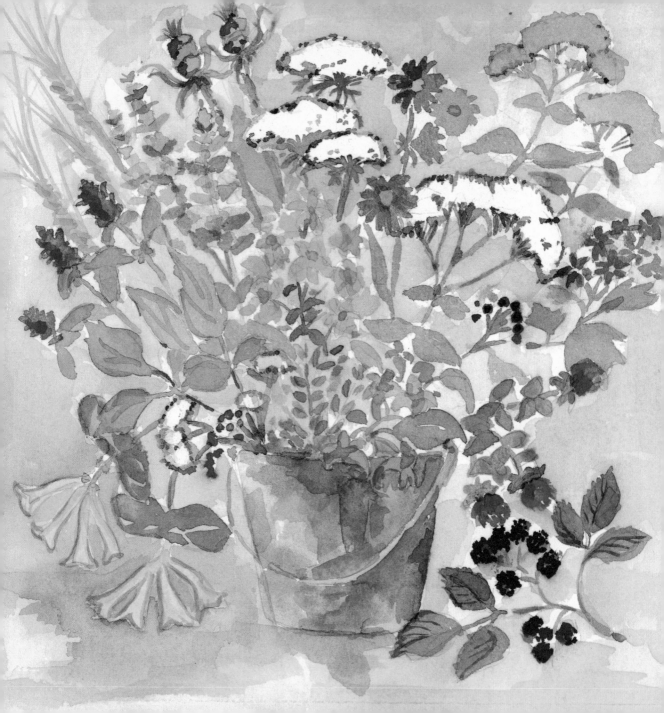

June

One clear morning just before the Summer Solstice, I drive up to the cabin to look for ginseng (*Panax quinquefolius*) in the deep gap and to gather all-heal and elder-flowers to dry for our winter medicine chest.

The ginseng root isn't dug in June but is easier for me to locate now when it sends up its delicate white blossoms. My climb down into the gap is successful. I will remember the cool bank where it thrives and then come back in the fall when the roots are bursting with energy. I make my way up along the steep sides to a small sunny meadow between the ridges where the elder bushes cluster with their deep taproots finding moisture from a wide shallow summer run. They are in full flower. I stand still a moment enjoying their foamy beauty and full fragrance before I ask the elder mother if I can cut a few of her blossoms before I move on.

Tall wands of blue all-heal poke up through the grass with clouds of sparkles of white moths around them. I fill up the empty space in my basket with several long spikes and part the thigh-high grasses in a path back up the cove to the cabin.

Those grasses, the entire *Gramineae* clan, are the first plants to ripen, their grain plumes sending out seeds from now until late October.

1. Jewelweed; 2. Honey Suckle; 3. Ginseng; 4. All-Heal; 5. Oats;
6. Run Mint; 7. Teasel; 8. Queen Anne's Lace; 9. Chicory;
10. Joe Pye Weed; 11. Fireweed; 12. Blue Cohosh; 13. Red Clover;
14. Blackberry

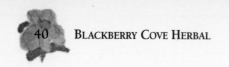

No wonder they are the most prolific plants in our climate! Before I turned off the blacktop onto the dusty mountain road this morning, I was nearly dizzy with the sweet smell of newly cut hay from every field along Mill Creek Valley.

The tall wild grasses I push aside are a mixture of species, but just as nutritious to the wildlife as the alfalfa or timothy being baled for winter cattle. The variety I randomly pick for identification turns out to be a wild oat, *Avena fatua*.

This afternoon I had planned to do some repairs on the cabin where flying squirrels had nibbled the wood siding—just like Hansel and Gretel, I think.

But the air is so still and the mid-day sun so hot, it is as though I am under a Midsummer spell. I sit nearly motionless in the clearing for several hours, lulled by the sun, intense and tropical. Bright light streams through the mature forest canopy in powerful golden shafts, not a leaf moving.

Solstice is that moment when the sun stands still. Midsummer June is a luxuriant green achievement when all the frantic rush of spring culminates in this long pause at the top of the year. My head tells me that tomorrow the great wheel will begin its long slow diminishing of light into fall and winter, but at this hour my heart is in that timeless realm of Faerie where sunlight never dims, inclement March is only a faint memory, and this honeysuckle fragrance is forever.

Only when the sun begins to slant a little through the trees do I stir, still hot and sluggish with perspiration in salty beads above my lip. On impulse I stick my head under the pipe of flowing springwater near the cabin, and then plunge my whole body under. A cold jolt back to reality!

The nearly undetectable evening breeze that curls down the mountain is still warm as it dries my skin and coaxes my vision back into focus on ox-eye daisies and bright purple thistles (*Cirsium vulgare*) blooming by the cabin steps. Yellow rays of St. John's wort (*Hypericum*), the most magical herb of all on Midsummer Eve, have turned toward the western sun and lead my eyes with them down the lane.

When I bend to pull on my shoes, I see a pair of antique gold eyes watching me solemnly from a dark and squat little body. It is a toad, our common American toad (*Bufo terrestris*). This one is only about two and a half inches long, and it would be easy to mistake him for a rock. His is just the color and bumpy texture of the weathered round limestones in the cove—down to the irregular lighter splotches across his back.

We watch each other for a few seconds while I remember the grandmother stories about how the toad represents the spirit of stones. He is the guardian of those great and terrible powers within the Earth herself. According to Appalachian mountain wisewomen, we won't learn all those secrets by science alone, but by listening to the spirit voice that speaks from the rocks that form the very body of our planet.

Because the toad is the ancient keeper of so many mysteries, mountain ruffians as well as gentle folk desired its powers. Our ancestors believed inside every toad's head was a beautiful and precious jewel. When old toads die they lose this treasure, which then turns to a dark stone with the toad shape of its former owner etched on it. These "toadstones" give protection from evil and bring good health to their owners. If you leave a small gift or silver coin outside for the fairies on Midsummer Eve, they will lead you to a toadstone.

A dried toad heart prevents thieves from being caught. One gruesome old way to prevent bad luck is to hang nine toads upside down to die. But white witches know that all cruelty to living things comes back threefold on the perpetrator.

If you meet a toad, something good and lasting will soon come into your life. If you make friends with a toad and place him carefully in running water at midnight, you will become a toadwoman. Toadwomen can speak with the animals and have great sex appeal!

I wish my toad friend well, but I am not waiting around until midnight. I load my gear and my basket of herbs in the jeep and reluctantly leave Blackberry Cove again.

My grandparents' deserted farmhouse is not far from where the mountain road comes into the paved state road. Without thinking about it, I turn up the lane. Several of my elderly uncles still keep the house weatherproof, mow the grass, and make hay from the fields to store in the old barn.

Between the icehouse and the cellar is the grassy slope where I found my first four-leaf clover. Tonight while I sit here in the long twilight of this most magical night, with familiar and deeply loved ghosts all around me, I find another.

The four-leaf clover brings good luck. There are faded four-leaf clovers pressed between the pages of my books and painted on my jewelry and china. I collect four-leaf clovers, I give them away, and I do have good luck.

When I was a child I spent long warm summers with my grandmother and grandfather on this farm making gold-fringed memories. The family was a big one, with my mother nearly the eldest of twelve children, plenty of grandchildren, farm animals, dogs and cats, and wide meadows with clumps of mysterious secret woods.

But it didn't offer a little girl much individual attention. Grandmother Lulu Catherine was the busy matriarch running the place, plus the Methodist Church and the Democratic Party in Mill Creek Valley. Grandfather Osa was a mild gentleman who wore a hearing aid, usually switched to "off."

My memory vividly conjures up one afternoon when I was about five. Grandfather and I had been pottering, and we eventually ended up sitting near this very spot. He picked an ordinary clover and asked me, "Can you find one of these with four leaves?" I reached over and picked one, two, three. His eyes flew wide, he jumped up, grabbed my hand, and hauled me in to my grandmother.

"We have a Finder!" he shouted on the way in. She put down whatever she was doing in the kitchen to see my little bouquet of four-leaf clovers. "We have a Finder," they said in chorus. I puffed out my chest and glowed. It was my proudest moment! One of the cousins might be the pretty one, an uncle the smart one or musical one, but I was the Finder.

When the aunts sat outside slowly fanning themselves on light summer evenings like this one, my grandmother or my mother would sometimes say to the others, "She's a real Finder. Watch." Then to me, "Honey, go find a four-leaf clover." With that kind of motivation, more often than not, I brought back a four-leaf clover or two. I was completely sure of myself. I was a Finder.

A Finder brought pride and honor and good luck to the family, and everyone on that porch knew it. Grandmother read her King James Bible every day, but she also believed in ghosts and tokens and four-leaf clovers. She was Scotch-Irish and Welsh and, of course, Celtic, the backbone of Appalachian culture.

Someplace in the mists between the mountains of Scotland and the mountains of West Virginia the family had misplaced its knowledge that a Finder of four-leaf clovers could see the fairies and foretell the future. A Finder was blessed with second sight, like someone born with a caul.

My love of plants and the details of nature was with me from the beginning, but that recognition from my clan set it as unalterably as the patterns of a leaf.

Driving home this evening I listen to a radio interview with an author about ethnobotany. His new book is about traditional plant uses that are being lost in the Amazon.

"That is what I am," I say out loud. "An ethnobotanist!" But my tribes are Celtic and Teutonic and Appalachian and West Virginian.

As an herbalist and writer my passion has been finding those green tendrils curling through my own culture and place. I have stalked the few remaining old-time herbalists in the hollows, spent hours over musty books, and let the plants and mountains themselves whisper their secret language to me.

My own culture was once nature-centered. People particularly observant and respectful of the natural world were valued and rewarded. Everyone understood it was important to live in rhythm with the seasons. So even now in our postindustrial age, somewhere inside all of us the old aunts and uncles are tugging, and we feel a little uneasy. If we are cut off from the green and the rain and the cycles, our spirits wither.

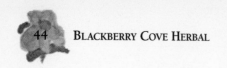

I believe it is within the depth of our own heritage and place that we each will ultimately find the clearest vision of our relationship to the natural world.

Now that humankind's very survival depends upon this harmony, we must all become Finders, looking for the magical four-leaf clover.

Ginseng

Deep in the coolest of coves in June our native "sang" lifts its small foamy umbel of white with filaments like untwisted silk. It is the *Panax quinquefolius* so highly prized in Chinese medicine and becoming so rare in our mountain woodlands.

The spot where I find and gather ginseng has a distinctive fragrance of rich leaf mold rarely warmed by direct sunlight. It is so steep I slide most of the way down and then climb slowly back up again. I identify a particular ginseng plant in June, mark it with a stake, and then dig up the tuber in late October. Some years I find only a single plant or two, so I just enjoy the beauty and leave them alone. This year I found a little grove of young ginseng plants and one that had matured enough over several years to send up three leafstems. I will harvest the fat yellow tuber just before winter when all of the plant energies are down in the root. It will be a good tonic for my family this year.

This fresh root is pleasantly sweet to the tongue with a bite of characteristic bitterness. A mountain tradition is never to touch the ginseng root with anything made of iron.

The Chinese prescribe it chewed or infused in wine or water for chronic stomach or lung problems and for all ailments associated with old age. It is said to be a sedative to "animal spirits" as well as an aphrodisiac. Folk wisdom says ginseng is wasted on the young. Save it until you are old.

Our Western scientists have discovered that ginseng is rich in vitamin D. It will raise low blood pressure and seems effective in lifting depression. The most common use is to treat weakness or exhaustion by increasing vitality.

Here is the traditional method to use ginseng. Put a teaspoon of grated fresh root or 1/2 teaspoon of dried root in a cup of water and simmer gently for ten minutes. This should be taken once a day as a tonic or three times a day for a specific condition.

Korean Song in Praise of Ginseng

The branches that grow from my stalk are
three in number, and the leaves are five by five,
the back part of the leaves is turned to
the sky, the upper side downward.
Whoever would find me must look for a
great tree.

All-Heal

All-heal (*Prunella vulgaris*) blooms all summer in the cove, but in June the tall spikes are like wands of brilliant blue flames. I gather them now at their peak of intensity. Every bit of the plant above ground can be used either fresh or dried. I hang the whole spikes upside down in the cabin to dry. When they are "chip" dry in several weeks, I strip the leaves and flowers from each stem and store them in a close-fitting tin.

All-heal is a common weed with a huge family of cousins. Only a few are native to these hills, and like most of them, *Prunella vulgaris* was brought from the Old Country. Maybe it naturalized from hay brought to feed sheep or cows during the Atlantic sea voyage, and maybe a grandmother brought it in a leather pouch to cure her family's wounds.

All-heal is part of that great labiate order of plants. Flowers grow on tall stems sometimes called "ears" (like corn). They don't all bloom at once, and the stems

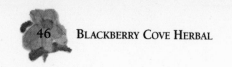

themselves are rough and hairy, so the plant is often ragged looking. It throws out lateral roots, and at every point a new plant springs up. In the middle of sunny pastures the stems are only a few inches high, but along the shadier edges, the stems can grow two feet tall.

All-heal has always been highly esteemed by herbalists. Its other folk-names are heart-of-the-earth, blue curls, hook-heal, slough-heal, and brunella. The last comes from the German *Brunnellen* because it helps to cure inflammation of the mouth and throat called *die Breuen*.

There is not a better herb for curing inward and outward wounds, say the grandmothers.

Steeped in honey, it is used to dab on ulcers in the mouth or cold sores on the lips. Combined with rose petals and taken as a tea, it is used to cure headaches. All-heal tea is a general internal strengthener and a good gargle for sore throats. An old-fashioned treatment for piles is to take an all-heal sitz bath.

The traditional method of making all-heal tea is to pour a pint of boiling water on a small handful (1 ounce) of dried herb. Steep ten minutes. For use internally, take a wineglass full a day.

This is an herbal charm from the mountain grandmothers to heal a broken heart. Cut out a little heart from blue material. Fill it with all-heal and white rose petals. Add a copper coin to attract a new love. Stitch it up with white thread, and wear it next to your heart from one full moon until the next full moon.

Oats

The wild oat growing in the cove is *Avena fatua*, only one of about twenty-five cousins of the domesticated *Avena sativa*. It is the great-grandmother of grains—symbol of the Greek goddess Demeter. Both the fruit and the stems or "straw" are used by country grannies to cure everything from bedwetting to skin rashes.

By late June the tall blonde leaves ripple in breezes and are plump with their milky substance of nourishment. They have been so important in healing and nutrition because the prolific grains can be used fresh or dried and stored as groats for use by people and livestock all winter long. The fat grains are rich in carbohydrates and proteins but quite low in fat. They have significant amounts of calcium, iron, phosphorus, the B vitamin complex of thiamine, riboflavin, niacin, and folic acid, and vitamins E and K.

A weak watery oatmeal or gruel is the traditional remedy for fevers and upset stomachs of every cause. Oatmeal is not soluble in alcohol or oil, but in a thick paste made with water, it is a natural emollient for skin rashes.

The grandmothers say oatmeal and oatstraw tea will give you strong bones, an even blood sugar level, a clear circulatory system, and steady nerves. They prescribe an oatstraw bath to ease hemorrhoids, and oatmeal for breakfast to encourage even granny's appetite for sex.

Oatmeal face scrubs are now sold commercially and oatmeal soaps and bath powders are in the most expensive bath shops. But it is so easy to make your own for pennies.

Wild oatstraw is easily gathered in midsummer and hung to dry. Store it as whole as possible in brown paper bags. Nearly every whole foods grocery store carries oatstraw today, and of course buying commercial organic oatmeal is much easier for most of us than gathering the straw or grains.

Here are some Appalachian recipes:

Oatstraw Tea

Pour a quart of boiling water over a cup of oatstraw and steep for ten minutes. You can take almost unlimited amounts of this.

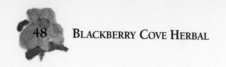

Oatstraw Bath

Add two quarts of reheated oatstraw tea to a bathtub full of very warm water and soak in it for as long as you like.

Oatmeal Bath

Tie up a handful of dried oatmeal in a washcloth to soak in a tub of warm water with you. Squeeze the wash cloth occasionally so the milky juice swirls around in the water. Rub the washcloth over your skin. This bath will soften your skin and relieve itches.

Oat Tonic

This is granny's remedy for an upset stomach. Pour two cups of boiling water over a cup of dried oats. Let stand an hour. Pour through a cloth and wring the juice out. Mix with a little honey if you like. Take by the spoonful as often as you can.

Have oatmeal for breakfast and make oatmeal cookies. And hang up in the kitchen someplace a handful of oats tied up with red string, while saying three times:

Oats, oats,
Green or groats,
Soothe and heal
With every meal.

Honeysuckle

In June the country lanes winding to Blackberry Cove are sultry with the scent of honeysuckle. It binds up the tangle of green entwining the rusted wire fences, and then cascades over the top with creamy flowers. The air hangs rich with a sweetness both innocent and hinting at our deepest, most sensual inclinations.

Mountain preachers warn that the windows of young girls' beds should be closed on these hot honeysuckle-sweet nights lest the air itself conjure up erotic dreams.

Some mountain families say it is bad luck to cut honeysuckle and bring it into the house. It might give you a sore throat or diminish the second cutting of hay.

But matchmaking grandmothers bring in armloads to fill china vases or tuck into bouquets of roses. They know honeysuckle in the house will bring a wedding in the family within the year. And they know that honeysuckle (or woodbine—another old name for it) is the symbol of true love. Chaucer's faithful lover

Wore chaplets on hir hede
Of fresh wodebind, be such as never were
To love untrue, in word, ne thought, ne dede
But ay steadfast.

Lucky young men find "honeysuckle sticks" to carry when they go courting. These are hazel sticks around which the honeysuckle has wound itself. They are beautifully twisted when the honeysuckle is unbound.

Our native honeysuckle here is *Lonicera sempervirens*. The rampant woody stem twists around anything in reach, and the elongated leaves are nearly evergreen in our hills. The early summer flowers often have a tinge of orange and have deep spurs like the columbine. In fact, our native red mountain columbine is sometimes called "honeysuckle" by country people.

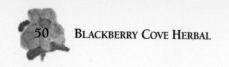

Mountain children pick the flowers of both plants, nip off the base with their teeth, and suck out the sweet nectar.

Honeysuckle dropped out of the pharmacopeia when trained physicians stopped using it in the mid-nineteenth century. "Doctors have left honeysuckle to the hedgerows, and rightly so," declared the French physician Roques in 1837. Country grandmothers have continued to use honeysuckle–and rightly so. Now we know it is rich in salicylic acid (the essential ingredient in aspirin) and has some antiseptic properties, and we can conjecture about more attributes.

Once upon a time a grandmother from the deepest hollow between the tallest mountains would cure jaundice with the true honeysuckle. She chewed the fresh leaves into a paste and rubbed them on her patients' foreheads while saying some prayers, but no one remembers the prayers any more. Maybe you can still hear them on the wind in the deepest hollow between the tallest mountains.

Honeysuckle Flower Tea

The grandmothers know the flowers gathered at the full moon, dried and made into a tea, are good to soothe winter coughs. Pour a quart of boiling water over a cup of dried flowers and infuse for ten minutes. Take two cupfuls a day for a tickling cough.

Honeysuckle Leaf Tea

Gather the leaves in the spring at the waxing moon just before the vine flowers. Use fresh or dried. Pour a quart of boiling water over a half-cup of dried leaves or a cup of fresh leaves. Infuse ten minutes. This is said to be particularly good for sluggish bowels.

<u>Honeysuckle Root Tea</u>

Gather the honeysuckle root in the fall at the dark of the moon nearest the first frost. Dry it or use it fresh. Boil a quart of water and a half-cup of chopped roots for two or three minutes. Let it stand for ten minutes. Take a cup a day as a general tonic, say the grandmothers.

St. John's Wort

The most magical herb of all in Blackberry Cove is also the herb-of-the-day in popular culture. It is St. John's wort. *Hypericum perforatum* is the tall and showy Old World variety that grows so freely wild in the cove, but two native species grow there too. The little *Hypericum ellipticum* blooms in moist places along the run, and *Hypericum punctatum* with its distinctive black lines claims a sunny spot in the meadow.

By the Summer Solstice around June 21 all three have bright yellow five-petal flowers. If you hold a petal up to the sunlight you can see little translucent red spots or "suns." These actually contain the potent St. John's wort oil.

Its name *Hypericum* is Greek and means roughly "over an apparition" because the sun-loving plant is so powerful against evil spirits that one whiff will drive them away. The "wort" part of St. John's wort is actually an old Anglo-Saxon word that means a medicinal plant. Some other country names are amber, devil's scourge, penny john, touch and heal, hundred holes, and witch's herb.

The grandmothers say St. John's wort will lift an evil spell. Physicians today have found a St. John's wort regimen to be quite effective in treating depression. Depression certainly feels like an evil spell! The grandmothers won't tell us about melatonin and serotonin and all the chemical components of clinical depression, but they have told us for thousands of years that cheerful yellow St. John's wort will make us optimistic and content again.

I won't go into the myriad ways the medical profession is recommending the use of St. John's wort. You can find that everywhere from the supermarket tabloids to the Internet. I will share with you, though, some very old traditional Appalachian uses of the highly respected St. John's wort.

The grandmothers say the most potent St. John's wort is accidentally found with a glad heart. Gather and hang bunches over the doors at midnight on Midsummer Eve to banish evil spirits and protect the house and barn. Cut St. John's wort at noon on Midsummer Day to use for curing an ailment.

St. John's wort sprigs should be worn tucked in clothing near your left armpit to guard against black witches and enchantments. Here is a St. John's wort charm repeated by some Scotch-Irish grannies as they gather the herb.

St. John's Wort, St. John's Wort,
I envy whoever carries you.
I pluck you with my right hand.
I carry you with my left hand.
Whoever finds you in the cow pen
Will never be without kine. (an old word for "cow")

Eligible girls can hang up St. John's wort above their beds on Midsummer Eve to tell if they will marry within the year. If the branches are still fresh next morning, they will marry for sure.

If you accidentally step on St. John's wort after sunset on Midsummer Eve, you will be carried away by a fairy horse and not let go until the sun comes up.

The grandmothers say St. John's wort tea relieves pain, removes the effects of shock, and is a general tonic for the mind and body.

St. John's Wort Tea

The flowers and leaves on the flower stems should be gathered and then dried as fast as possible.

Pour a cup of boiling water over three teaspoons fresh or one and a half teaspoons dried herb. Infuse for ten minutes. Drink up to a cup three times a day.

St. John's Wort Salve

Steep a handful of fresh St. John's wort flowers in a cup of olive oil for a month. Strain. It will be a beautiful clear red!

Melt beeswax slowly in the top of a double boiler and gradually add the St. John's wort oil until it reaches the consistency you like. Pour it into a jar and let it cool.

This salve is a traditional remedy to soothe minor burns, sunburns, and wounds that are already closed and beginning to heal.

July

Dog Days are from mid-July to mid-August. Our ancestors noticed Canicula, the Roman dog star, was in conjunction with the sun—attributing mad dogs, irritable shedding snakes, and all sorts of vile behavior to Dog Days.

Ponds stagnate. Poison ivy thrives. The fetid air maddens us now with gnats, hungry mosquitoes, and flies, all of us enveloped in a humid miasmic cloud that hangs over these hills.

Tansy, our splendid dowager Shetland sheepdog, died last week just at the onset of Dog Days. She left our family still echoing her exuberant delight and that total loyalty only dogs know. And she left us with a great hole in our hearts. Tears still well up regularly, but I try to remember it was during these Dog Days thirteen years ago that she was born. I remind myself that at this moment, tiny Sheltie puppies are still carrying on that particular life-shape in this great varied universe.

Yesterday, on the third Sunday in July as usual, my mother's clan gathered at the homeplace on Mill Creek near Blackberry Cove for a picnic. It is that West Virginia institution called "The Family Reunion." Kin from just across the field and as far away as Philadelphia pulled up the dusty lane to unload covered dishes and children under the great sugar maples shading the faded white house with its wide porch. For as long as even the oldest of us can remember, we've been eating potato salad together in this annual communion of re-weaving our visible ties while our hidden spirals of DNA bring forth new generations of babies with Great-grandmother's blue, blue eyes.

Lunch is set out at high noon as usual. My mother Bessie's baked West Virginia ham is succulently resplendent, as always. (She goes to Maine with me every summer, orders ham from the local menu and sits back in wicked anticipation. "Hmph! A football ham. Probably boiled." She wouldn't dream of ordering lobster.) There is red velvet cake, Aunt Genevieve's creamy pink Jell-O pudding, and Aunt Lessie's great pot of green beans cooked to tenderness in bacon broth. The table stretches twenty feet. New generations have added Mexican dishes and exotic jewel-colored raw vegetables. In addition to the big jug of lemonade and the sweating pitchers of iced tea, there are now little bottles of Starbucks chilled cappuccino.

In that hot lull after dinner, the oldest uncle, Uncle Ernie, presides from the lazy porch swing while my mother and her sisters circle their lawn chairs on the grass in a crones' council. They worry about my father out there clanging horseshoes for hours in the hot sun. He is still the undisputed horseshoe-pitching champion, sustaining challenge by a dozen knights—some as much as sixty years his junior. I hear them consider the possibility that my daughter and her red-headed beau will get married this year, why a peevish uncle boycotted the picnic, and how my own scattering of gray hairs have finally reached critical mass.

The rowdy school-age kids are down in the crick netting minnows and turning over rocks for hellgrammites. Up at the house a bevy of exquisite young cousins sit on a blanket stringing little glass beads for ankle bracelets and to twine in their shiny hair.

The teenagers are off in a pack exploring the barn and the icehouse and the vine-covered rusted Ford pickup truck with 1959 license plates. The youngest of the kin is almost two. He is splashing in a melting ice chest and shouting "No" at every opportunity.

Just before the food is laid out again for supper, the talk gets around to family history, as usual. Someone asks, "What year did Great-granddaddy Dennis die?" Uncle Ernie tells us, "We laid him to rest on Christmas Day 1942," painting a vignette of loss and sadness around the printed words on a genealogy chart.

When the heat starts to ease after supper, a cousin of my generation organizes a car convoy to the old cemetery several hollows away, over a twisty road two inches deep in dust, because "some of the younger ones don't know how to get there." We turn in at a farm gate generously nailed with "No Trespassing" signs, following the time-honored Appalachian custom that kin always have unquestioned access to the graveyards.

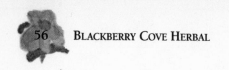

Someone has mowed around the crooked and nearly illegible eighteenth-century stones. We move slowly among them. Some of us crouch down to read the names. We eat the blackberries that hang fat and juicy from brambles in the cemetery.

July is my least favorite time at the cabin. It is too hot, too intense. I am overwhelmed. Not for me is this wild energy of July, in a beat of time so strong and relentless I would dance to exhaustion if I joined in.

It is the songs of plants growing and fruiting, of insects, the chitin-covered ones, clicking, fluttering, gnawing, sucking, preying, buzzing. Their own sounds are loud and insistent. Their short one-season lives belt a frenzied song to me as our energies converge, but I know I am not of their realm.

Chicory is blooming fiery blue. Queen Anne's lace and black-eyed Susans aren't even dusty yet beside the road. I see one perfect sphere of red clover blossom bobbing among the others. A honeybee is probing, buzzing, probing, buzzing.

The Appalachian grandmothers say bees go around humming their song of praise to the Earth all day long. It is very unlucky to kill a bee because they have in them the wisdom of the Earth and the spirits of fairies.

Mountain people say they should never be sold. Borrow or trade for a swarm of bees, and they will produce more honey.

Bees know secrets. They won't thrive near a household full of spite or ill will. The grandmothers believe bees tell news of family births, marriages, reunions, and even deaths. And they like to be told. A little of each dish served after a wedding or funeral should be set out for the bees.

When a bee flies into an Appalachian house, it is good luck, but the luck disappears if the bee is killed or chased out. Bees must leave by their own will.

A bee flying around a sleeping baby is bringing happiness and a pure heart. If a bee lights on you, money is coming. If you dream of a bee, you will soon come into your own—by position or the blossoming within.

There are strong ties between bees and beekeepers. Those of honest natures can walk through a swarm of bees.

Once upon a time there was a mountain granny who lived in the hollow just over the hill. She loved her bees so much she was always telling them things, and she said they whispered back. "If I have any wisdom at all," she said, "it's because of what the bees tell me." She would sit outside and sing a beautiful song in a language no one understood, and the bees would cluster all over her like she was a beloved Queen Bee. Five days after she died at the ripe old age of ninety-three, her neighbors walked to the top of the hill to lay flowers on her grave. They found it humming with her bees, singing her praises to the universe.

Chicory

Chicory is one of only two species of this native Old World plant, *Cichorium*. Its clear blue flowers decorate our roadsides and meadows in high summer, while the other is the cultivated garden endive.

The grandmothers know either one can be a powerful love potion when given by a man to a woman. Never try it the other way around, they warn!

One of the first wildflowers a country child picks is the pretty pink and blue, dandelion-shaped chicory blossom growing on its scraggly stem. And it is one of the first disappointments, because by the time the little hand-held posey is inside the kitchen door and given to mama, the flowers have wilted away.

Chicory also dries to nothing in hay, but it is good forage food for horses, sheep, and cows. Rabbits especially love chicory! I sometimes see them in the cove, nibbling the leaves, in the morning before the flowers open and then again in the late afternoon after they have closed for the day.

Some folk-names for chicory are succory, sun follower, bride of the sun, way light, blue sailor, cursed maid, and watcher of the road.

Once upon a time, some grandmothers say, the sun looked down upon a beautiful maiden with blue eyes and fell in love with her. He came down to earth to woo her, but she wasn't interested in him. He got so provoked that he turned her into chicory, who is destined to follow him all day with her blue eyes.

Once upon a time, say other grandmothers, an abandoned blue-eyed girl sat so long on the wayside waiting for her runaway lover that she turned into chicory. A few grandmothers say the young woman was such a scold that her lover had good cause to skedaddle. That is why chicory tastes so bitter.

It is that bitter taste that some of us love so much in our coffee. Chicory roots are gathered in the early fall and air-dried for a fortnight. Then they are ground to the consistency of coffee grounds, mixed in (as much as you like), and brewed with the coffee. Chicory adds a dark color and a distinctive sharpness to the flavor of coffee. It doesn't contain caffeine, but it does have a high silica content, and is said to soften the jolt of caffeine-rich coffee.

The grandmothers prescribe chicory tea as a laxative, to ease rheumatism, as a diuretic, and as a general tonic. This is the traditional recipe.

Chicory Tea

Boil a half-cup of dried and coarsely chopped chicory root in a quart of water for ten minutes. Strain. Drink a cup with meals.

Bruised fresh chicory leaves make a poultice that is cooling to skin inflammations.

The grandmothers warn that too much chicory taken internally can cause bad eyesight. A lotion made from the fresh flowers, though, is a soothing eyewash for irritated eyes.

Chicory Flower Water

Pour a quart of boiling water over a cup of clean, freshly picked chicory petals. Steep ten minutes. Strain and cool. Bathe eyes with the cool water as often as you like.

Queen Anne's Lace

Most of us consider Queen Anne's lace a noxious weed to be rooted from the garden, but in Blackberry Cove it is beautiful. The feathery green foliage looks too delicate to support its wide lacy umbels in July. But even after the wildest thunderstorm they are sturdy bouquets of white froth.

This is the wild carrot, *Daucus carota*, whose close Asian cousin of the same species is Peter Rabbit's fat orange garden carrot.

By August the flat flower heads have ripened their seed and curled up into a "bird's nest." The oldest grandmothers called it bird's nest, bee's nest, or just lady's lace (because Queen Anne wasn't yet on her eighteenth-century throne when they crossed the Atlantic).

All of the grandmothers, however, know it is a mysterious herb that wins love and has a "certain force to procure lust." On the first windy day nearest the full moon after the bird's nest forms, gather the flower heads. Rub them gently between your hands so the tiny black seeds fall onto a plate while the chaff blows away. Carefully store the hot peppery seeds to enliven winter soups and spice up your love life. Be careful, though, because the grandmothers whisper that it encourages conception.

Queen Anne's lace root dug in early fall and boiled in water is a traditional mountain diuretic. Boil a cup of chopped roots (dry or fresh) in a quart of water for fifteen minutes. Take a cupful a day to "provoke" urine.

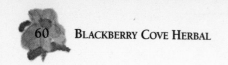

<u>*Sauerkraut with Wild Carrot Seed*</u>

1 16-ounce can sauerkraut
1 small onion stuck with 3 cloves
1 grated carrot
salt and pepper
1/4 teaspoon Queen Anne's lace seed
1/2 cup dry white wine
1/2 cup water

Rinse the sauerkraut in cold water. Place all the ingredients in a pan and bring to a boil. Simmer for an hour. Remove the onion and take out the cloves. Slice the onion and return it to the pan. Enjoy!

Jewelweed

Low on the shady side of the gap descending from Blackberry Cove to the river, jewelweed blooms from midsummer to early fall. After a summer shower or on a foggy dew-laden morning in early autumn, droplets sit like jewels on the leaves and flowers themselves. They refract the light in bright facets like the rarest diamonds, and there is no question about why we call it jewelweed.

It is also *Impatiens capensis*, the native annual whose cousins are the garish pink and red impatiens sold in garden center six-packs. Our jewelweed flowers are yellow and orange. They are variously marked and mottled with reddish brown, and their distinctive blossom is made up of three sepals, the lowest one sack-like and funnel-shaped.

Other country names are slipperweed, butter and eggs, snapweed, and touch-me-not. It is called American jewelweed in the British Isles, where it has naturalized in a reverse migration.

Appalachian children love to touch the ripe fruit capsule and jump back as it pops with great energy—sending out seeds several feet. The five thick stamens spring back in coils and tickle little fingers.

The grandmothers tell us that wherever poison ivy (*Rhus radicans*) grows, you are likely to find its natural antidote, jewelweed. They say if you are going to be around poison ivy, crush the jewelweed stems and leaves and rub the juice on your skin to prevent an inflammation. If you do break out with the poison ivy rash, jewelweed juice will soothe it and hasten the cure.

Jewelweed Lotion

Simmer a quart of crushed jewelweed in two quarts of water for ten minutes. Strain and cool. This can be stored in the refrigerator for a week. Rub the lotion on skin both to prevent poison ivy rash and to soothe it.

Appalachian grandmothers use fresh jewelweed juice to banish warts and make jewelweed salve for corns and ringworm.

Jewelweed Charm for Curing Warts

Say this three times while you rub fresh jewelweed juice on a wart.

> *Jewelweed, Jewelweed,*
> *I pray today*
> *That this wart on [Name]*
> *Will rot away.*

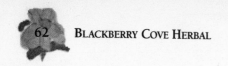

Jewelweed Salve

The traditional way to make this salve is to cook fresh jewelweed stems and leaves in melted lard for a few minutes. Then strain out the plant material and let the lard cool for use as a salve.

An alternate way is to steep a half-cup of chopped fresh jewelweed in a cup of olive oil for several days. Strain. Melt shaved beeswax in a double boiler and stir in the oil to a desired consistency.

Fireweed

This homely little annual weed (_Erechtites hieracifolia_) gets its name because you can often find it in profusion over newly burnt-out areas. In our cove, though, fireweed grows along the run in open places. It brightens the moist meadow with fuzzy little white flowers from July to nearly frost.

The grandmothers must have learned about fireweed early on from their Indian neighbors. They use the fresh leaves, finely chopped and laid on the skin, for eczema. These same chopped leaves can be macerated into a paste and applied directly to hemorrhoids or piles. In fact, sometimes fireweed is called pilewort.

Pilewort Tea

Pilewort tea is made by steeping one-half cup of the whole flowering plant (coarsely chopped) in a quart of boiling water for ten minutes. This tea is used to soothe a sore throat, ease hiccups, and to stay diarrhea.

Applied externally, this tea can be rubbed on like a lotion to help relieve muscular soreness.

The grandmothers say fireweed must be used fresh. Even the tea or distilled oil is useless if kept for more than a day or two.

Blackberry

The old forest at Blackberry Cove was cleared by a family named Poling over two hundred years ago. They carved out a little farm on the flat sunny ridges and treasured the sweet icy water from the gushing spring. My practical grandfather bought the abandoned overgrown farm in the 1920s to produce apples, peaches, and tomatoes for a local cannery. Then after his tragic death in the early 1940s, the orchards and gardens began to melt back into wilderness. By the time I was a young woman, the cove was a tangle of blackberry briars. In a few hours we could fill buckets with fat sweet blackberries for cobblers and jellies and for eating fresh with cream. My grandmother had even made blackberry wine when I was a child. But now the walnut and hickory trees have grown tall, shading out those first re-growth thickets, and we only find blackberries on a few sunny edges of the new forest.

They are our native *Rubus*. In spring they bloom a starry white, and by the Fourth of July we nearly always have the first berries.

The mountain grandmothers treasure these shiny black gifts from the mountain for their delectable flavor and their healthy properties. They say just crawling under blackberry bushes can relieve adolescent blackheads. If you gather your blackberries in the moonlight of July's full moon, they will protect you from "evil runes," whatever they might be. Some grannies would pass young children backwards and forwards three times through a blackberry bush to cure them of a hernia.

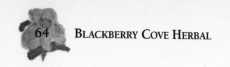

Here are two old charms to soothe a burn with blackberry leaves.

Apply fresh blackberry leaves to a burn and say:

> *There came three angels out of the East.*
> *One brought fire, two brought frost.*
> *Out fire, in frost.*

Take nine fresh blackberry leaves and dip them in spring water. Lay them against a scald and say three times to each leaf: The Maiden Bride came out of the East.

And don't forget, say the grandmothers, it is bad luck to eat blackberries after the Autumn Equinox around September 21.

The rootbark is a traditional mountain remedy for diarrhea. Gather roots at the dark of the moon after the berries have disappeared. Peel off the rootbark and dry quickly in a warm oven. One ounce dried root boiled gently for fifteen minutes in a pint of milk makes the decoction. Take a half teacup full every hour for diarrhea.

Fresh leaves can be dried anytime and used for diarrhea also. Infuse one ounce of dried leaves in a pint of boiling water for ten minutes. Take a little more than a half teacup full every hour, say the grannies.

Blackberry jelly improves circulation and attitude, they say. It has the opposite effect on the bowels as the rootbark or leaves.

Here is a very old recipe:

Blackberry Jelly

"Take the juice of blackberries and make your Sirrop of it to a pound of blackberries take a pound of sugar and put half the Sugar to ye juice and let it boyle, then put in the

blackberries and let them boyle as fast as you can take them off and Shake them oft put in the rest of the Sugar by degrees as they boyle but touch them not, when they are enough the stones will look clear. So you may do currants or cherrys."

Blackberry vinegar is a traditional remedy for a feverish cold. Here is how to make it.

Blackberry Vinegar

Gather the berries on a fine day, stalk them, put into an earthenware vessel and cover with vinegar. Let them stand three days to draw out the juice. Strain through a sieve, drain thoroughly, leaving them to drip throughout the day. Measure the juice and allow a pound of sugar to each pint. Pour into a pan, boil gently for five minutes, removing scum as it rises, set aside to cool, and when cold, bottle and cork well.

This is a mountain grandfather's recipe for blackberry wine.

Blackberry Wine

Mash two and one half gallons blackberries in a five-gallon crock. Add fifteen pounds of sugar and enough water to fill the jar to the rim. Put cheesecloth over the jar and let it work in a dark, cool place for about ten days. Then strain and put into a five-gallon keg. Lay the keg on its side and fill it up to the bunghole. As the pummies (the pomace or residue of crushed fruit) work out over the sides of the keg, add more water to keep the keg full. When the wine quiets down, close the hole with a cork with a rubber tube in it. Put the other end of the tube in a glass of water. Leave the keg like this until the wine quits sparkling and is still. Then close the bunghole tight with the spigot. Let the wine age for two or three months more. It will be ready to drink by the time cold weather sets in.

But we all enjoy our blackberries best in a West Virginia cobbler.

Blackberry Cobbler

5 cups fresh blackberries
1 cup sugar
3 tablespoons flour
2 tablespoons butter
2 cups flour
4 teaspoons baking powder
1/2 teaspoon salt
1/2 teaspoon cream of tartar
2 tablespoons sugar
1/2 cup butter
2/3 cup milk (about)

Butter an eight-by-ten oblong baking dish and fill it almost to the rim with blackberries sweetened with the cup of sugar. Sprinkle the three tablespoons flour over the berries and dot with butter. Set aside.

In a bowl sift flour, baking powder, salt, cream of tartar, and sugar. Cut in butter until mixture resembles coarse meal. With a fork, stir in enough milk to form a ball of dough. Turn out on a floured board and roll dough to one-fourth-inch thickness. Cover the blackberries with the dough and trim the edges. Cut a vent in the top to allow steam to escape during baking. Sprinkle the top generously with additional sugar and bake in a hot oven (400°F) for forty-five minutes or until the crust is browned and the juices bubble. Serve warm with rich cream.

August

It is late afternoon before I can get away to Blackberry Cove. This early August morning in Harpers Ferry was already steamy when I went out to cut a few dusty bunches of lemon balm. The air still smelled sweetly of dew, but the sky was that peculiar flat white that meant the day would be scorching. I gave up any thought of work.

By the time I had slowly puttered through a few chores, the whole village was dreamy with a haze of heat. I knew I wanted to get away to the cabin, to those violet blue mountains in the west, those great misted Appalachian foothills.

It is still summer, but the bend has decidedly curved toward fall. Nearly every plant has made its seed, those tiny packets of rich nutrients that are ready to fall or be carried away to rest in the dark until next spring.

We are all covered with a fine dust of weariness. There is still harvest work ahead, but we have begun the gathering and can sense the coming quiet time.

Rich heavy air blows in the jeep window, but it's too hot to dry damp hair blowing around my face or cool my shirt sticking to the seat. Before long though, the flat valley lifts to tranquil views of hilly little farms and deep woods. My heat-heavy spirits lift too, with the sight of the tall teasel and Joe-Pye weed blooming along the narrow road.

A silvery veil of moisture has already settled on the pasture in front of Grandmother Lulu's deserted white farmhouse as I turn into the dirt lane. The winding little road leads nearly eight miles over mountains and through twisting gaps before it comes to the river. Grandmother Muriel's house sits tucked up against a steep cliff with the Potomac River within earshot across the field in front. Blackberry Cove is back up in the hills, almost a mile away.

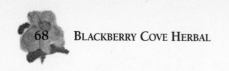

But today I pull in past the old mailbox at Grandmother Lulu's for a while before going on over the mountain to the cabin. I sit on the porch hoping the afternoon will cool, but I know it won't on this night. The bed under the metal roof will be as hot as an oven. I remember how I lay there as a child, covered with sweat until sleep came over me.

I sit here remembering those long evenings of my childhood. After supper, in the dreaming twilight, my aunts and uncles drifted slowly in the porch swing or gently creaked on the glider. Sometimes it was nearly too hot to talk.

Eerie balls of blue light would sometimes quietly rise above the field out toward the crick. They would float along near the marshy ground before disappearing as suddenly and mysteriously as they came. We called them jack-o'-lanterns, and I later learned they were swamp gas self-igniting when the conditions were right. They were lights carried on these hot dark nights by the spirits of the swamp themselves.

A brown rabbit with long ears is out for supper at the edge of the field, barely visible among the long shadows. Her ancestors reminded our first Appalachian grandmothers of the great hares of old Europe and gave them comfort.

The hare is sacred to the Earth Goddess of rising suns and fertility. Mountain witches, whisper the grandmothers, can turn themselves into rabbits and run all night in disguise. Only a silver bullet can bring them down.

In the hill country if you meet a wild white rabbit, it's unlucky because they are the soul-shapes of young girls who died of grief after their lovers left them. If you meet a brown rabbit, it is good luck, although you really should go home and start your journey all over again. Well, too late for that!

Some say dreaming of rabbits means watch out for secret enemies. This bad luck attributed to rabbits and hares, I believe, grew out of the notion that rabbits were associated with evil witches. Actually, they are sacred animals, a sign of happiness and renewal—beloved by the wise grandmothers. They say dreaming of rabbits means you can look forward to discovering a mystical trail to spiritual and material treasure.

Once upon a time such a wise old grandmother lived just over the next hill. She was a good round woman who knew her herbs, and her neighbors called on her for healing and advice. Some folks called her a witch, but she was always good-natured. She said, "Truth is truth. You'll know me by the fruits of my deeds."

One day a tall skinny preacher with a puckered-up mouth came along the cove to her cabin. The grandmother was in bed with a sore leg.

"I have come to name you a witch!" he declared. "I saw a rabbit in my garden last night, and I shot it with bits of a silver button. It ran off limping and squealing. Everyone knows a rabbit will turn back into a witch–still shot. And here you are in bed!"

"Foolish old man," said the grandmother. "Don't you know when you hurt an animal, you hurt yourself? It is true that I was hurt by your bullet last night, but not in the way you think. I took the injuries myself that should have been yours because I knew you were a silly man without any sense about the secrets of life. But since you came to claim what is yours, I can't help you."

When the grandmother got up from her bed as fit as a fiddle, the preacher ran off down the road in a tizzy. After he was out of sight, and the dust had settled, she set off to find the rabbit.

It came limping up to her, and she took it home and nursed its wounds.

The old preacher fell flat, on the way home, and broke his leg. The grandmother went to him with her herbs, and gradually his leg got well again.

He never shot another creature, and any time he heard anyone call the grandmother a witch, he would shush them and say, "There are many secrets in life we know nothing about."

As for the grandmother, she got on with her healing. Sometimes when the night was clear, her spirit would run with the rabbit and know what it was like to be young and limber again.

It is nearly dark and still hot when I finally pull up in front of the cabin. Most evenings a cool breeze drifts down the mountain just before sunset, but not on this sweltering day.

Water is barely dribbling out of the pipe near the cabin, so I walk up to the old sugar maple with the spring at her roots. I hear a loud "plop" as I lift the lid to the basin where the water collects, and out of the corner of my eye I see a fat frog jump into the cool darkness. I can smell the sweet limestone water. The level is lower than usual, but there is still more than enough for me and the other creatures in the cove.

By the time I unpack and settle on the deck, the only light I see is the moon rising over Owl Mountain, burning slowly in the hazy sky. Tomorrow early I will gather Joe-Pye weed and red clover because it will be another hot day in Blackberry Cove.

Joe-Pye Weed

Huge, graceful Joe-Pye weed (*Eupatorium purpureum*) weaves its rich purple onto Blackberry Cove's late summer loom of goldenrod and blue asters. It stands far above them—nearly five feet tall, giving rich texture to these moist meadows.

When I gather the giant clusters of tubular florets that make up the round-topped flowers, a lovely scent of vanilla fills the air.

It is the fresh roots, though, that the grandmothers use as a diuretic, to discourage kidney "gravel," and as a generally strengthening tonic. They must have learned about its healthful use from their Native American friends and relatives. In legend, Joe Pye was the eighteenth-century woodland Indian who first taught European settlers about this glorious native herb. Some other folk-names are gravelroot, trumpet weed, jopi weed, boneset, hempweed, and queen of the meadow root.

The fresh root is the part traditionally dug at the dark of the moon in early fall.

This is how the grandmothers use it. Simmer a fresh root the size of your little finger in a pint of water for ten minutes. Drink one-quarter cup, warm, every hour as a diuretic. Drink a cup a day, warm or cold, as a tonic or to resist "gravel" if you have a propensity for it.

Teasel

Teasel (*Dipsacus sylvestris*) came with our ancestors from Europe, and, like it, we have each found our niche in this mountain landscape. Our teasel grows in the old field near the road at the end of summer. Its delicate purple flowers are mixed with spine-like bracts that make the whole head a sort of pincushion. Dozens of these cones rise up to six feet above each plant. It is a near relative to the *Dipsacus fullonum*, which is still grown commercially in England. That cousin just has a little more crook on its spines.

The grandmothers cherish teasel in their dooryard gardens alongside other old-fashioned herbs like tansy and yarrow, which have also slipped under the fence to scatter in the fields.

After the lovely purple flowers fade, the dried heads are placed on spindles and revolved against newly woven cloth to "tease" it. That means it raises a fuzzy nap, making the fabric more soft to the skin. So it gets its folk-name teasel. The grandmothers also sometimes call it bath of Venus.

Some say sore eyes can be soothed with the rainwater that puddles in the hollow cups of mature teasel. Other grandmothers whisper a cure for warts on your hands. You should wash your hands three nights in a row under a round moon with the stagnant rainwater that collects in the leaves at the base of the teasel bracts. The warts will disappear before the next full moon.

I savor teasel's late summer beauty in the cove. And I gather the tall stately teasel in honor of its beauty and its usefulness to our kind. It graces our home in fall flower arrangements and in our Christmas decorations.

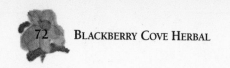

Run Mint

I think the mint in Blackberry Cove is *Mentha spicata*, but I can't be sure. Regardless, we call it run mint because it grows right alongside the run in a moist spot barely dappled with sun.

Mints are the despair of botanists trying to classify them. They have been culti-vated and crossbred for thousands of years in the Old World, where the Romans brought them to northern Europe from the Mediterranean. Then they were brought here, continued to cross, and escaped from the garden to the field, where they cross-bred with our one native species that is itself quite variable.

Our mint stands about a foot tall and has toothed leaves with no stalks. The summer flowers are small, delicate, and lavender-colored. The dark, shiny leaves look cool even on a hot day. When those leaves are brushed, they give us that familiar clean and refreshing fragrance.

I hang it in bunches on the screen door, where it discourages flies and is fragrant every time the door opens. The grandmothers say mice hate the scent of mint! In the hottest part of summer every room has a big vase of fresh mint leaves.

Herbalist John Gerard wrote about mint at the turn of the seventeenth century that "the smell rejoiceth the heart of man, for which cause they used to strew it in chambers and places of recreation, pleasure and repose."

The grandmothers know mint tea is not only flavorful but will stop hiccups and windiness (flatulence), as well as "giddiness of indigestion"—upset stomachs. Babies with colic are sometimes given a mild mint tea.

Some grandmothers recommend a bath in mint water to soothe hemorrhoids. Others say mint tea will bring down a fever.

Summer potato salad with a light sprinkle of freshly chopped mint leaves is mys-teriously delicious. If the grandmother has a little Welsh in her background, she might cook her cabbage with fresh mint leaves.

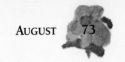

Of course, we all know how good fresh mint tastes with lamb. Mint jelly and mint vinegar are good, too.

In fact one of mint's folk-names is lamb mint. Some other names are Our Lady's mint, green mint, spire mint, sage of Bethlehem, fish mint, Frau Munze, and mackerel mint.

Mint Vinegar

Bruise fresh mint leaves and fill a quart jar loosely with them. Fill up the jar with white vinegar. Cover and let stand in a cool dark place for fourteen days. Strain and bottle.

Mint Sauce for Lamb

Take a cupful of mint vinegar, add a pinch of salt. Heat it just before boiling. Pour over a cup of chopped fresh mint leaves. Let it steep ten minutes. Stir in three tablespoons of brown sugar.

Blackberry-Mint Jelly

Take a cup of blackberry jelly, and mix into it two tablespoons of fresh finely minced mint leaves.

Once upon a time gypsy caravans traveled through these hills and camped in the summer fields. One day a gypsy woman came up to a house where the lady suffered terribly from hay fever. She looked around the garden and said, "You have the cure right here. Pick some fresh mint every day and put it in a muslin bag. Tuck it inside your pillowcase and inhale the scent while you sleep. Also wear it around your neck in the day." The sneezing lady did, and she was cured.

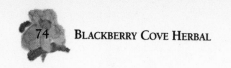

Red Clover

One of the prettiest late summer sights in Blackberry Cove is the red clover (*Trifolium pratense*) bobbing in the tall grass. Each rosy ball is often topped by a bee while several others hover nearby. Clover blossoms are the favorite of bees, with that heady fragrance so reminiscent of the juice from rich purple grapes.

Deer love clover too, and it is good forage for domestic browsers like horses and cattle. In fact one folk-name for red clover is hart clover. Other names are sweet clover and plaster clover.

Our red clover grows up to three feet tall. The leaves are much larger than those of the little white clover in the cove. Sometimes those long oval leaves are marked with a distinct V.

Red clover blooms all summer here, and like so many of our common wild plants, it was brought from Europe—probably in hay for domestic animals.

The first grandmothers must have been delighted to find it growing in their newly cleared meadows, and they knew exactly how to use it.

A plaster for hot swollen joints is made from clover heads. Some mountain grandmothers use this same ointment to rub on painful abdomens.

Red Clover Ointment

One cup freshly picked flowers steeped in one cup melted lard (or warm olive oil) for twenty-four hours. Strain out the clover. Heat lard or oil again and slowly stir in shaved beeswax until you get the desired consistency.

The whole upper part of clover can be used, but the flowers are the best part. All of the plant is dried by hanging bunches in a warm dark place.

Clover tea has a pleasant flavor, and the grandmothers prescribe it for indigestion or flatulence.

Red Clover Tea

Pour a cup of boiling water over one-half cup of freshly picked clover blossoms or one-quarter cup of dried clover heads. Steep ten minutes. A teaspoon of honey can be stirred in after the cup is poured from the teapot.

Red Clover Eyewash

This is a favorite to soothe red irritated eyes.

Pour a pint of boiling water over one-half cup fresh flowers. Cool. Bathe eyes with the cool clover water. Keep in the refrigerator and discard the unused part after several days.

Clover Bath for Melancholy

Take one handful of red clover blossoms and one handful of chamomile flowers. Simmer in a quart of water for five minutes. Cool a little. Add a half-cup of new milk. Pour this mixture in a bath of "blood warm" water and get in for a long soothing soak.

Back in the hills some grannies use dried clover blossoms to scent their pipe tobacco or snuff. Dried blossoms are also placed among linens (much like lavender) to impart a pleasant fragrance.

Of course, finding a four-leaf clover is always good luck! Some grandmothers say a green salve of four-leaf clovers (made with secret words) can make you invisible when it is rubbed over your entire body. For it to work, you can't miss a single wrinkle! All the grandmothers agree that carrying a four-leaf clover can (if the season and the moon are just right) let you see the fairies.

Once upon a time two young sisters were walking home across the fields from their auntie's house. The sun was just going down below the hills in the west, and a round red moon was just coming up over the hills in the east.

"Look at those little white lights twinkling up that hollow over there," pointed the little sister.

"What lights?" asked the big sister, peering up the hollow.

"Look. Can't you see them? Little people are carrying lanterns . . . some are dancing. Can't you hear them laughing?"

"No!" cried big sister as she grabbed little sister by the hand and ran lickety-split for home.

When little sister was pulled in the door and had told her story to the family, her mother put her to bed right away under the thickest quilt. While Mother was brewing up a cup of boneset tea for little sister, Grandmother carefully looked over little sister's muddy shoes.

"That's it!" she exclaimed. "There is a four-leaf clover stuck to the sole of her shoe."

Blue Cohosh

This stout native perennial grows on the deep moist forest floor of our cove where the tallest trees make a thick canopy. In late spring when blue cohosh (*Caulophyllum thalictroides*) blossoms, sunlight sparkles down on the dainty yellow six-pointed stars, but by late summer the blue "berries" are in full shade. They are not berries at all, but simply the seeds themselves that have burst open the ovary to form a fleshy blue outer layer.

Each stem has only one leaf, divided so it looks like many leaves. Although blue cohosh can grow nearly four feet tall, in our mountain forest it barely rises over eighteen inches. The root (rhizome really) is the treasured medicinal part of the plant.

Some other folk-names of blue cohosh are blueberry root, blueberry cohosh, blue sang, papoose root, squaw root, and yellow sang.

Traditionally, it is during a waning moon, between the time "berries" form and the first hard frost, that the fat root is dug, washed, and slowly dried in a warm dark place for several weeks.

The Appalachian grandmothers learned to value and use blue cohosh from their Native American neighbors and kin. Powdered root was used with great skill by woodland Indian women to induce menstrual flow and to hasten and ease the pains of childbirth. All of the grandmothers warn: Never use blue cohosh in any form until the last few weeks of pregnancy.

Several slices of dried blue cohosh root boiled in two cups of springwater for five minutes makes a bitter-tasting tea that the grandmothers prescribe for colic, sore throats, cramps, and coughs. The usual dose is a quarter of a cup several times a day.

You can even use the warm tea, whisper some grandmothers, to bathe and ease sore private parts.

Today we know blue cohosh is rich in minerals like potassium, magnesium, calcium, and iron. I don't harvest and use this beautiful woodland plant myself, but every time I encounter it, I nod a silent "thank you." Blue cohosh eased the pain and fear for many of our foremothers when other paths were not open to them.

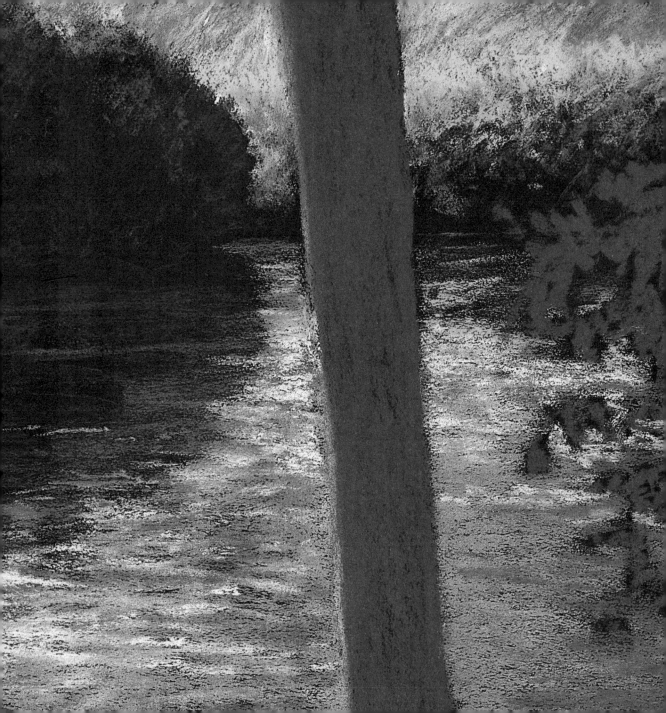

Autumn

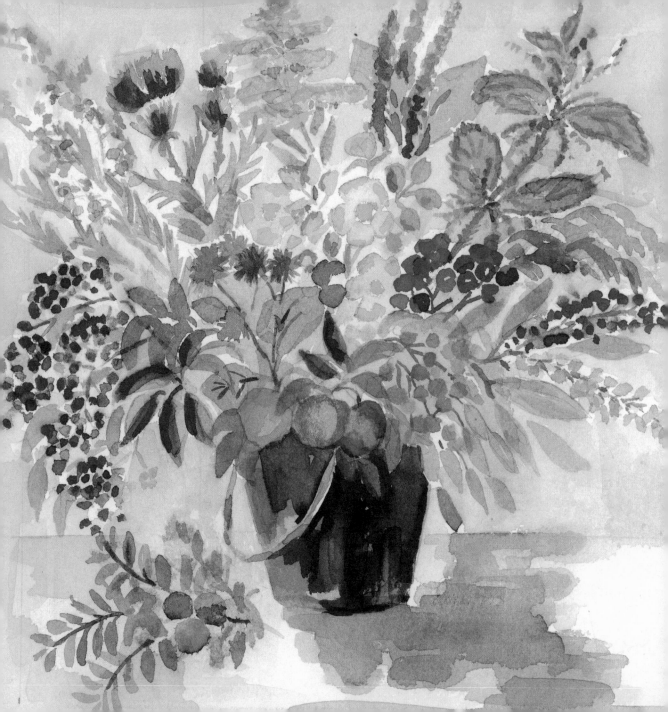

September

September in Blackberry Cove is golden. The warm yellow sunlight on my face this afternoon makes me drowsy as I doze outside the cabin, feeling the slowing down of life between these hills. Weightless threads of thistledown and tiny dandelion tufts are flecks of suspended gold in this quiet afternoon light. A drift of goldenrod draws my eye, recalling Thoreau's description of it as "spilled sunshine."

Summer's urgency has overflowed. It has seeped into roots and seeds, and we can nearly hear this sound of trust as Mother Earth herself leans back, sighs deeply, and says, "I've done all I can do this summer. Let autumn commence."

So I stir from this four o'clock rest, bring out my yellow legal pad, and start making a list of harvest priorities. I will be gathering and drying herbs in earnest now for my own family and friends and to sell at the great Waterford Fair early in October.

Frost is still nearly a month away here in these Appalachian foothills, but September brings the first chilly mornings. This morning will be nearly over before the cool heavy dews have dried enough for gathering leafy herbs.

I hear the distant honking of geese in these early hours. Although they are flying down the Potomac River valley only a mile away, the sides of the cove are too steep for me to see them.

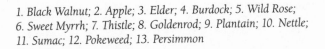

1. Black Walnut; 2. Apple; 3. Elder; 4. Burdock; 5. Wild Rose;
6. Sweet Myrrh; 7. Thistle; 8. Goldenrod; 9. Plantain; 10. Nettle;
11. Sumac; 12. Pokeweed; 13. Persimmon

I listen for as long as I can to their ancient song of fall migration. The grandmothers say the goose is a holy bird that flies in front of the Earth Mother. Her large flat feet were made by working the treadle of a spinning wheel, spinning out the strands for the web of life. Freya, the powerful Norse Mother Goddess, was often portrayed as goose-footed. So it is with a deep sense of awe that I witness this flight of Canadian geese, sisters to the magical Mother Goose of our foremothers.

I cut tall plumes of sweet myrrh (*Artemisia annua*) from along the fenceline today. Its strong, spicy smell is September itself to our family, and the jeep will carry this fragrance well into winter. Staghorn sumac torches grow intermingled with the myrrh, so I cut several bunches while I am at it. They are already turning red, one of the first blazes to light the fall countryside.

Tomorrow I will be busy gathering sage and rosemary from the fenced-in herb garden in Harpers Ferry, but today I am enjoying this dreamy woodland pace. Clusters of wild sweetbriar rose hips are delicate elfin fare compared to the big round ones of *Rosa alba* in the town garden, but I gather them because their delicate flavor will make a jelly fit for Queen Maeve herself.

A whole grove of paw paw trees has grown up in the cove in the last decade or so. Even their huge buttery leaves can't hide the fat paw paws hanging down this time of year, so I carefully gather a small basket of the soft-skinned fruit to eat and use right away.

It is only when I no longer feel the warm sun on my back and start to wonder where I have left my sweater that I realize these golden hours are drifting into evening. The back of the jeep can't hold another branch of anything, and Tansy is giving me her unblinking gaze that says it's time for dinner. It will be nearly a year, next July, when Tansy slips away forever. Although I cannot see into the future, I cherish each day with the gentle old dog. I close up the cabin, put her bowl of food down on the deck, and finish up the last half of my peanut butter sandwich.

When I close the gate at the end of the lane, Blackberry Cove is already in shadow. As we drive up and out of the cove, it is still bright along the dusty road when it flattens out, winding in and out around the ridges, past the old one-room schoolhouse. This evening sun is directly on it, lighting up the new coat of red paint it recently acquired as part of its transformation into a hunting camp. It was seventy years ago that my mother, her eight brothers and three sisters, attended Number Six School on the Stringtown Road.

"The boys swore they saw a woman in a long white nightgown following us, in the trees, up on the bank above the road when we walked to school in September. She would appear, disappear, and then appear again," my mother told us. "But we girls never saw her."

Was she the White Goddess herself? The poet Robert Graves reminded us of our common and deeply rooted reverence for the female powers of creation. Were my uncles, as little boys, just trying to scare their sisters, or did they see and feel, as children often do, a spirit of our grandmothers? The woman was clothed in white, the color of mystery and death to our ancestors in the northern forests of Europe. Was she our Earth Mother herself—first harbinger of autumn, foretelling the dying year?

I keep an eye out for this woman in white, but the only white I see is the drift of asters along the road. These tiny flowers bloom at the Fall Equinox in September, and as children we were told not to eat blackberries after the Michaelmas daisies bloomed because the devil had spit on them. By September there is not a blackberry left in the cove, so I feel safe.

Tonight billows of starry asters catch the last sunlight over these hills, twinkling with gold as I turn out onto the highway.

Elderberry

"Summer isn't here until the elderberry bush blooms, and it doesn't end until the berries are ripe" is an old mountain adage.

Those little trees (or big bushes) are a beloved familiar sight in our Appalachian countryside when they bloom with masses of creamy fragrant flowers. Then by late summer those wide flat flowers have turned into drooping bunches of juicy purple-black berries. If you want those berries in our cove, you have to be quick, because the birds love them, too.

Elderberry (*Sambucus canadensis*) bushes are cherished for their beauty, fine taste, health-giving properties, and wise magic. The ancient Romans made a musical instrument like panpipes from the hollow stems. They called it a "sackbut"–hence the Latin name *Sambucus*.

Anglo-Saxons called elderberry trees *aeld*, hence "elder." *Aeld* meant fire. The hollow stems were used as pipes for smoking various herbs and to puff oxygen on a dying flame. Some other common names are black elder, pipe tree, bore tree, hylder, eldrum, and elhorn.

Just a generation ago every country child knew elderberry stems made great pop-guns.

Farmers never cut elderberry brush from along their fencelines, and gypsies never cut or use elderberry wood in their fires.

The Appalachian grandmothers revere the elderberry bush and use nearly every part of it to heal nearly every sort of ailment. They know the Elder Mother lives in each bush and watches over it. It is bad manners ever to cut elder wood or take the flowers or berries without asking permission from the Elder Mother.

The grandmothers say an elderberry bush near your house protects your family from misfortune, particularly from getting struck by lightning.

An elderberry stick carried in your pocket protects you from rheumatism, a twig is very good luck in a bridal bouquet, and two twigs tied in a cross with red thread and hung over the barn door protect the animals inside. Gather elderberry leaves on the last day of April and hang them over your doors and windows for protection from ill will. If you have a lingering illness, go to the nearest elderberry bush on a moonlit night and ask politely to be cured. Elderberry stakes will last as long as iron. If you switch a child with an elderberry wand, the child will stop growing. Rub a wart with an elderberry leaf and then bury that leaf. When the leaf rots, the wart will be gone. If you sit under an elderberry bush on Midsummer Eve, you will see the King of the Fairies. Don't sleep in the shade of an elderberry bush, or you might get caught in dreams of Elfhame and never return.

Once upon a time, up in the deepest hollow in the deepest valley, a young man made a beautiful cradle for his unborn child. He fashioned it out of thick white elderberry branches for strength and decorated it into beautiful fanciful curves with slender pliable elder twigs.

When he laid his newborn son in the cradle on a soft brown rabbit skin, it commenced to cry and cry inconsolably. Its little legs jerked every which-way, and the wee baby was actually lifted right up in the air several inches and let fall back down.

The kindly old midwife, who was still in the cabin tending to the new mother, came running and snatched the baby up in her arms.

"Go outside right now," she directed the young father. "Go to the Elder Mother in the tree where you cut the wood for the cradle. Take off your hat, bend down on one knee, and tell her you are sorry you cut her wood without permission. Tell her about the beautiful cradle and about the sweet new babe. Say, 'Elder Mother, you gave me some of your wood. I will give thee some of mine when it grows in the forest.' Ask protection for the child all his days. Then be silent and listen carefully. If you hear only silence, you will know she has blessed the cradle and the baby."

The young man did just as the grandmother told him. After that, the baby slept peace-fully in the cradle with a little smile on his tiny pink lips. And he was happy and kind and loving all his days!

The elderberry bush has been called the medicine chest of country people. Every part except the root and bark is used in healing, and the root and bark can be used for a black dye.

Leaves are traditionally gathered to dry in June and July on a fine day after the dew has dried. Fresh leaves can be gathered any time.

Elder Leaf Ointment

The grandmothers use this to rub on bruises and sprains.

3 parts fresh leaves to
4 parts lard

Heat slowly together until the lard is green. Strain through a linen cloth, and use when warm.

Modern Variation of Elder Leaf Ointment

Combine equal parts leaves and warm olive oil. Let stand until oil is green. Heat again gently and add shaved beeswax until you get the desired consistency. Cool and use. This can be used as an oil too, without adding the beeswax.

Elder Leaf Water

The grandmothers use this to bathe sore eyes and "snuff up your nose" when you have a head cold.

Boil a cup of fresh elder leaves in a quart of springwater for ten minutes. Strain and cool.

Remedy for a Headache

Put fresh elder leaves on your forehead or temples and lie down in a dark room.

Collect elder flowers when they have just opened. Elder buds are useful too, so gather these at the same time. The lovely flowers and buds are best when used fresh, but they can be dried quickly—in a warm oven with the door ajar—to be used all year.

Elder Flower Lotion

Fill a gallon jar or crock with fresh elder flowers and buds, pressing them down. Fill it with two quarts of boiling springwater. When it has cooled a little, add an ounce of moonshine (or vodka). Let it stand in a warm place for three hours. Let it cool in a chilly place like a springhouse or the refrigerator. Strain and bottle.

The grandmothers say this clears up nearly any skin problem.

Elder Flower Tea

For colds and flu, go to bed and drink elder flower tea as hot as possible. Heavy perspiration and refreshing sleep will follow, say the grandmothers.

Cold elder flower tea is a good spring tonic to be taken every morning from April 1 to June 1, before breakfast.

Without the sweetener, elder flower tea can be used as a lotion to bathe sore eyes. It can be applied with a linen cloth for boils and skin irritations of all kinds.

Method: Pour one pint of boiling springwater over one handful of fresh flowers or half as much dried elder flower. Steep for half an hour. Strain. Sweeten to taste with honey.

Elder Flower Vinegar

This is good on salads, as well as being a traditional remedy for sore throats.

Fill a quart jar with fresh elder flowers. Fill it up with white vinegar. Let steep in a cool dark place from full moon to full moon. Strain. Bottle and use.

Elder Flower Ointment

This is good for burns or scalds and as a cosmetic cream. Elder flower ointment is particularly good for sores on horses, say the grandmothers.

Infuse a handful of fresh or dried flowers and buds in a cup of warm lard or olive oil for twenty-four hours. Strain. If using olive oil, warm again in a double-boiler and add shaved beeswax until you get the desired consistency.

Elderberry juice has supreme power to ease everything from colds to asthma, diarrhea to dropsy and everything in between, insist the grandmothers. "It even dyes silver hair black," they say. "But why would anyone want to give up a silver crown?"

My own Grandmother Muriel made elderberry wine for years from the berries that hung from bushes along the river. Taken before bed, hot with sugar, it is a winter cold remedy.

Elderberry Wine

For two gallons of wine, use one gallon of elderberries. Boil in six quarts of springwater for half an hour. Use a long elderberry stick to break up the berries. Strain through a fine sieve. Boil again with six pounds of sugar. Let this simmer for half an hour. Cool. Stir in a teacupful of yeast. Cover it up. Let it work. After two days, skim off the yeast and put in a wine barrel. When it quits hissing (in about two weeks), stop up the bunghole. It will be ready in seven weeks and will keep seven years.

Elderberry Syrup

The grandmothers say this is good for promoting natural excretions of sweat, urine, and stool.

Pick a pint of thoroughly ripe berries. Stew them until soft in a cup of springwater. Strain. Add a pinch of powdered ginger and a clove. Simmer again for a few minutes. Strain again. Add as much sugar as you like while it is still warm. As this tastes delicious, just use it for enjoyment over pancakes or ice cream!

Use your favorite recipe for berry jelly and just substitute elderberries. Jars of elderberry jelly grace every grandmother's pantry shelf like a row of dark jewels.

In our house, we keep a tin of dried elder flowers to toss in a hot January bathtub for the ultimate luxury—a bath with the essence of summer in our mountains.

Wild Mugwort

Our wild sweet mugwort near the cove is *Artemisia annua*, the only annual in this large family of plants. Very generally, the artemisias are divided into three groups: mugworts, wormwoods, and southernwoods. French tarragon stands alone as the artemisia used for seasoning food.

While this fragrant mugwort, locally known as sweet myrrh or Sweet Annie, doesn't grow in Blackberry Cove proper, it is prolific just down the mountain along the river and railroad tracks. The first grandmothers probably brought seeds from the Old World for magic and to use as a vermifuge—to rid their family members and animals of internal parasites. Eventually this mugwort, like so many other plants, naturalized in our countryside.

Sweet myrrh must have been named after the precious Biblical myrrh given to the Christ child by a wise man because of its strong aromatic smell. In September there is no mistaking the plant. Nearly five feet tall in places, its delicate light green leaf-branches blossom in tiny, nearly invisible flowers and send a fine dust of golden pollen into the air with the slightest breeze. The whole plant is almost unbelievably fragrant!

It is easy now to forget its violent history as a powerful purgative for people and livestock. Both the mammals and the internal worms were made violently ill, but because the mammals were bigger, they usually survived while the parasites perished. It was a dangerous and inexact process, so even the most traditional grandmothers eschew it today when gentler methods are available.

We cut branches these early autumn days to hang and dry for winter arrangements. Years ago I filled a barn with drying sweet myrrh to make dozens of fragrant wreaths for the great Waterford Fair, but now my fingers have protested with twinges of arthritis. So I make just one grand wreath to grace our home with wild beauty and the heady smell of fall itself.

And I like to remember the magical heritage of this fine mugwort. There is an old belief that wearing a mugwort crown (or even a sprig in your lapel) at Midsummer Eve will drive away last year's disappointments and bring good luck in the coming season of growth. It restores weary travelers when they wear a leaf in their shoes!

Some mountain grandmothers still call it "muggins" for its old use of adding to a mug of ale. They say if you nibble a leaf in May, it will protect you from consumption, physical exhaustion, wild beasts, and paying too many bills.

> If they would eat leeks in March
> And mugworts in May,
> So many young maidens would not
> Go to the clay.

Staghorn Sumac

In September our Blackberry Cove sumac (*Rhus typhina*) presents its elegant crimson candelabras, those grand clusters of berries that grow atop the inconspicuous but plentiful little trees of our thickets and waste places. We don't even notice when they bloom reddish green in late spring, and we ignore the scraggly tree all summer. But by fall sumac is a starlet!

Sumac first draws our eyes now with these great staghorns of fruit, and by October the leaves are as intense orange-red as a sugar maple.

Several years ago when I was traveling on a train outside of London, I was enjoying glimpses of those exquisite little English gardens tucked behind nearly every house. I kept seeing a small tree, obviously planted as the focal point and carefully mulched all around. Eventually, it was with surprise and amusement that I realized it was sumac—the very native weed-tree we curse and wrestle out of our gardens. Then I looked at the profusion of yellow primroses growing wild on that English railroad embankment and thought about how every spring I carefully plant primroses in my Harpers Ferry garden where they almost never come back. Exotic or mundane is all in the perspective—"one man's cup of tea," and all that.

The first grandmothers must have marveled at sumac and learned how to use it from the first Americans. Now they know the leaves and bark can be used to tan leather, and the roots, bark, and berries are medicinal.

The bark can be gathered at any time, the roots are traditionally dug in late fall, and of course the berries are gathered as they ripen from July through early October.

A strong decoction of the dried or fresh root has been used for treating diarrhea and to bring down a fever. Powdered dried root is mixed with springwater to form an antiseptic poultice for "old sores."

Only gather the newest dark red cones of berries because sometimes the older ones harbor a plethora of little spiders. One grandmother advises gathering the berries before the rain washes off the fuzz. Never pick the poisonous variety with white berries!

Sumac Berry Tea

Pour a pint of boiling water over a handful of fresh berries. Steep for ten minutes.

This was once used to treat diabetes. A cupful a day can be taken to alleviate diarrhea, say the grandmothers. The cooled infusion is also good, they say, as a gargle for a sore throat and as a wash for ringworm or "tetter."

Sumacade

If you want to make sumac "lemonade," or sumacade, just for fun and because it is refreshing on hot September days, here is the recipe.

Bruise two cups of berries in one quart of springwater until the water turns pink. Strain twice. Refrigerate or serve over ice with sugar or honey to taste.

<u>Mulled Sumacade</u>

When the September evenings get chilly in the hills, try this:

Gently heat four cups of sumacade, three cloves, one stick of cinnamon, half a cup of brown sugar, and one sliced lemon for fifteen minutes. Don't boil.

Pour over a jigger of rum in a little cup. Sip and enjoy!

Thistle

Thistles grow as tall as we are in the little pasture by the apple tree in Blackberry Cove. They are the biennial *Cirsium vulgare*, inadvertently imported from the Old World by our ancestors, and they are indeed vulgar. Rough, ragged, and invasive, they still emit a bewitching nobility. Their great purple blossoms are breathtaking in early autumn.

My mother, Bessie, like a good farmer's daughter, scolds every year, "Cut down those thistles or they'll take over the place." Some years she has actually whacked them down herself!

Country people sometimes identify fertile farmland, though, by the thistles on it.

Once upon a time a blind man from several ridges over went with his son to buy a farm for the young man. When they got there the blind man said to his son, "Now keep the horses away from the thistles."

"I don't see any thistles," said the son.

"Well, then," said the blind father, "we'll just go on home. This land is too poor to buy."

Ours resembles the Scotch thistle, emblem of Scotland and the badge of the House of Stuart. The Scotch-Irish grandmothers would have recognized and loved it as soon as the first small rosettes sprung up in their new mountain homeland. At the death of James III of Scotland in 1458, his shroud was embroidered with "thrissils."

Herbalist John Gerard wrote more than a hundred years later that the thistle is "set full of most horrible sharp prickles, so that it is impossible for man or beast to touch the same without great hurt and danger."

In fact, the Scots' reverence for the thistle is said to have originated when a stealthily invading Norseman stepped on a thistle rosette in the dark of the night, let out a howl, and alarmed the sleeping Scots.

Sometimes it is called spear thistle because its strong spikes and sturdy shaft made a wicked spear. Now mountain children call thistles "blow balls" when the flowers go to seed and form downy white tufts. They even have a game in which they blow the puffs away, saying:

Mary, Mary, what time of day?
One o'clock, two o'clock . . .
It's time we were away.

The number of hours counted depends upon how many breaths it takes to blow them away.

Another old name is thistlefinch. We fill our finch feeders today with thistle seed, but there are few finer sights than a whole flock of tiny yellow goldfinches fluttering in ecstasy among the airy white whiskers of thistle heads.

Some grandmothers call it boar thistle and contend it is full of protective magic. A thistle head worn on a string around your neck is great protection from danger and will make you "merry as a cricket."

They also say a strong decoction of thistle leaves regularly applied to a bald head will restore hair. Thistledown has been used to stuff pillows, and the fleshy receptacle at the base of the flowers was once commonly cooked and eaten as a vegetable much like an artichoke.

Thistle leaves can be cut on a sunny day just before the plant blooms. They should be dried in a warm dark place and stored as whole as possible.

Thistle Leaf Tea

Thistle leaf tea, say the grandmothers, strengthens memory, helps circulation, eases most digestive complaints, and expels worms. Here is how to make it.

Pour a pint of boiling springwater over a handful of carefully crushed dried thistle leaves. Steep for ten minutes. Take by the wineglass full several times a day. May be sweetened with honey.

Paw Paw

We never had paw paws in Blackberry Cove until a few years ago. One spring I noticed a foot-high seedling with huge leaves right beside the lane to the cabin. The next spring it had doubled in height, and the following year it bloomed with that big exotic maroon flower. Two more seedlings appeared.

Now we have our own little paw paw patch producing several fat fleshy fruits every September. I watch the green paw paws swell all summer, but the Blackberry Cove possums usually get to the smooth tropical-looking fruit before I do. If my timing is perfect I am rewarded with a light green, eight-inch-long peanut-shaped paw paw just beginning to turn yellow with a few dark speckles.

Broken in half and eaten fresh from the tree, the scooped-out paw paw fruit is a juicy delicacy on our eastern side of the Appalachians. Paw paws are more prolific along the Ohio River—even though we have a community actually named Paw Paw right here in Hampshire County.

Delight in the sweet rich taste isn't acquired! Either you like it or you don't. If you can't appreciate that custard-like texture and rich heavy flavor right off—you never will. But for those of us who relish it, nothing can compare!

The botanical name *Asimina triloba* comes from a long-forgotten Indian word that French traders pronounced "asiminier." Botanists Latinized it to *Asimina*, and *triloba* refers to its two sets of three-lobed flower whorls. The name paw paw must also have been a Native American word.

The grandmothers say paw paw fruit soothes heartburn and is sure to relieve constipation.

The skin is too astringent to eat. It will make you pucker like a green persimmon. But the ripe paw paw flesh is good in any recipe as a substitute for bananas. Although the taste isn't at all like bananas, the similarity in color, texture, and use was noticed by our ancestors, who gave it many of the other common names: false banana, back-yard banana, poor man's banana, and West Virginia banana.

Paw Paw Meringue Pie

1 cup paw paw fruit mashed (without seeds)
1/4 cup sugar
1/3 cup flour
3 eggs
1 cup milk
1 cup cream
1 pie shell already baked

Combine flour and sugar. Add beaten egg yolks, milk, and cream. Mix well and add paw paw fruit. Stir over low heat until it thickens. Cool a little.

Make a meringue by beating the egg whites until stiff with three tablespoons of sugar and a pinch of salt. Pour paw paw mixture into the prebaked pie shell and spread with meringue. Bake at 350°F until the meringue is lightly browned (about thirteen minutes).

While the pie is baking, sing this mountain ditty:

Where, oh where, oh where is Susie?
Way down yonder in the Paw Paw patch.
Pickin' up Paw Paws, puttin' em in a basket
Way down yonder in the Paw Paw patch.

Wild Rose

In the cove we have but one kind of wild rose, *Rosa eglanteria*, whose tangle of sweet-briars grow just up the slope from the old apple tree. The most delicate of pale petals appear in June, and then they are gone again with the first wind, as fleetingly mysterious as Titania herself.

At high summer the dense thicket of prickles is not only a safe bower for the fairies, but also a secure nursery for baby rabbits.

It is in early fall, however, that the tiniest orange-red rose hips appear. I cut graceful canes to include in bouquets of autumn flowers, and I gather enough of the rose fruit under the full harvest moon to make a magical marmalade.

Rose Hip Marmalade

Bring one cup of rainwater and two cups of sugar to boil in an enamel saucepan. Simmer for four minutes to make a thin syrup. Add two peeled, cored, and diced wild apples and two cups of diced rose hips. When the mixture begins to boil again, cover and simmer for thirteen minutes. Stir occasionally. Strain through a coarse strainer and return to the saucepan. Simmer gently for three minutes, stirring constantly. Pour into the smallest sterilized jars you can find, and seal them tightly with this charm:

> *Tiny roses where wee folk sleep*
> *Your goodness is now bottled to keep.*

Cover the jars with a quarter-inch of melted beeswax if you want to keep them longer than a month.

This elixir should be savored on the finest white biscuits cut out with a thimble. Enjoy it when you need a quiet pause to let a little fairy magic back into your busy days.

Roses have been grown and cherished by the grandmothers since before anyone can remember. The dark red petals have been distilled into rose water, cooked up into sweet conserves, and dried for fragrant pillows or potpourris. Every sort of pink or white or yellow rose has been planted by every sort of doorway to bring pleasure and delight.

But the wild roses, say the grandmothers, carry the strongest rose energy for healing and love. If you can catch the elusive wild rose petals, dry them quickly in a warm dark place or use them fresh.

Rose Petal Infusion

This is good for headaches—particularly those caused by a head cold, say the grandmothers.

Pour a cup of boiling springwater over a handful of fresh or dried rose petals. Steep ten minutes. Add honey to taste.

Wild Rose Leaf Tea

Pick rose leaves on a sunny day after the dew has dried. Spread them in a single layer in a dry, dark place until they are "chip" dry. Store in a tin.

Pour a cup of boiling springwater over one tablespoon of dried, crushed leaves or two tablespoons of fresh, crushed rose leaves. Steep for ten minutes. Add honey if you like.

The mountain grandmothers recommend this for soothing sore throats and sores inside the mouth. It tastes surprisingly good!

Of course, today we know roses, hips in particular, are very rich in vitamin C, the universal cure for and preventer of colds. A single cup of rose hips has more vitamin C than a dozen oranges.

And roses are the ultimate symbol of love. Rose petals are strewn in the paths of brides and showered on honored leaders, and roses are given to our lovers as tokens from the heart.

The grandmothers say that the luckiest children are blessed by fairy grandmothers who stroke their soft faces with wild rose petals and whisper:

Sweet Baby, we give you this rose.
We have taken off the thorns today,
But we know that we can't take the
Thorns from your life.
So we bless you that your life, like this rose,
Will be beautiful in spite of its thorns.

Goldenrod

Goldenrod put on a spectacular show this year! By September the summer's wrenching drought had reduced our gardens and meadow margins to withered dusty patches. Then, one morning I turned the corner, and out of the river-bottom fog blasted a stand of gleaming goldenrod in full bloom, its yellow plumes glowing with drought-defying exuberance.

While it is goldenrod's propensity for brassy scene-stealing that draws the wrath of allergy sniffers, the true culprit is pollen-spewing little ragweed. Very little goldenrod pollen is carried by the wind. Butterflies and bees pollinate the flowers. By sunny afternoons in early autumn goldenrod is quivering with honeybees, providing a lovely tang to wildflower honey. Actually, our grandmothers knew a cup of goldenrod tea was just the cure for a stuffy nose or clogged sinuses.

Nearly a hundred species of goldenrod (*Solidago*) grow in the United States, and just one is native to Europe. Only the most dedicated botanist could classify them, and the promiscuous goldenrods like to cross-pollinate, causing even more confusion to our linear-thinking scientists.

All the members of this big gregarious *Solidago* clan are lovely, and at least one member, *Solidago odora*, is mildly anise-scented. There are giants up to eight feet tall and low-growing varieties in New England only a few inches off the ground. *Solidago sempervirens* is a seaside goldenrod at home both in salt marshes and on sand dunes. The goldenrod in Blackberry Cove is *Solidago canadensis*, the common roadside variety of West Virginia.

The word *Solidago* means "to strengthen," and the plant was held in great respect by early herbalists. John Gerard from seventeenth-century England tells the tale of speculators who shipped a whole boatload of dried goldenrod from the colonies to London when prices were at a premium. Just as their boat docked, the little English goldenrod called farewell-summer was found growing profusely in Hampstead Wood just outside London. The price immediately fell to nothing!

Goldenrod's herbal uses are nearly as numerous as its varieties. The blossoms chewed slowly are an old remedy for sore throats. A poultice of the roots is an Appalachian remedy for toothaches, and infusions of the leaves and flowers are used to relieve fevers, chest pains, urinary obstructions, and dropsy. The blossoms brewed into a lotion are a mountain cure for relieving bee stings and painful swellings.

Here is the granny woman's traditional recipe for goldenrod tea:

Goldenrod Tea

5 to 6 fresh or dried goldenrod flowers
4 cups boiling water
honey to taste

Strip the flowers from their stems and place in a warm teapot. Cover with boiling water and steep ten minutes.

A more sophisticated short-term herbal remedy for sinusitis is herbalist David Hoffman's brew:

Herbal Remedy for Sinusitis

1 part echinacea
1 part goldenrod
1 part goldenseal
1 part marshmallow leaf

These are brewed into a tea steeped for ten minutes. The inhalation of the steam is also recommended to relieve sinus congestion.

Goldenrod flowers make a good yellow vegetable dye, and the plumes dry well for winter flower arrangements. To use the flowers ornamentally or in tea, hang them upside down in a dark, dry place for several weeks.

I am feeling quite fortified this chilly dawn, with goldenrod tea steaming in my morning cup. I must admit, I stiffened it up a bit with a teaspoon of brisk Darjeeling while I pondered how things might be different if Virginia's fortunes had been made with goldenrod instead of tobacco.

October

October in Blackberry Cove is high energy! The leaves themselves are fiery. Maples zing with the most intense orange while the climbing vines of Virginia creeper and poison ivy come in next, spiraling up the bloodred oaks and golden ashes. My eyes are pulled relentlessly from one blaze of color to another, around and around the cove, up and up until an electric blue sky gives them the final jolt.

A flame-tailed fox squirrel just off the edge of the steps rustles through the ground leaves and darts up the elm trunk with her treasure of hazelnut or acorn. She is so intent on her task of storing up for winter, I can almost reach out and touch her.

My rocking chair on the deck looks inviting and warm in the sun, but I can only sit a minute before I am up and tacking the loose screen back down on the door. Then I check the height of the stack of seasoned apple logs for firewood, and I am off up the back path to the spring again to make sure there aren't any more leaks in the pipe.

We all feel it, this driving energy of October that carries an edge of fear. I don't depend any more on my garden and field to keep me fed through winter, but I still feel a little anxious, driven to make sure the cabin is tight for winter, driven to hoard—drying more herbs and buying more pumpkins than I can possibly use. A song of "It's now or never!" sings through my blood as loudly as through the sap of dying maple leaves, the tiny arteries of the squirrel, and the veins of the great deer who leaped across the road on this bright midday, plunging effortlessly up the mountain.

It was a magnificent Virginia white-tail buck with wide antlers. At most times of the year here in the cove these deer are only out in abundance on the edges of the day, morning and evening. But this urgency of fall brings them out under the noonday sun.

I think of Herne, the ancient horned hunter who was often portrayed as the stag. Mythology tells us he promised to protect us through the dark months of winter.

In these Appalachian woods the deer hunters will soon be enacting this ancient bloody rite of bringing down the Lord of the Wild Wood and providing meat for the cold of the year. I don't suppose many of them consider hunting season in this way, and the reality of slaughtering these graceful creatures is repugnant to many of us, but for a brief week or two these modern men reconnect with the old stirrings.

Even the October smells at Blackberry Cove are sharp. Fallen leaves have a crisp acrid fragrance as clearly recognizable to us as apple pie. Here in the midst of ridge upon Appalachian ridge of decaying leaves, it is pure in its pungency. I am conscious of breathing, savoring the smell and becoming aware of how it fills me with energy.

Sounds ring clear in the cove when the October morning fogs evaporate and the air is dry again. The decrepit old cricket sounds like an elephant in the dried brush, and the low trickle of the run is as loud to me as a spring torrent. When my cousin coonhunts on these moonlit October nights, you can hear his bluetick hound for miles.

It reminds me of how my little Scotch-Irish grandmother could best hear the crying baby up Fox's Hollow this time of year. She told the story over and over again every fall, and then my mother repeated it in the same way when my grandmother was gone. Mountain people like to repeat, I think, and like the familiar rhythm of words and thoughts going round and round.

Fox's Hollow is the next one down the valley from my grandparents' house. It was the hollow where my aunt would gather bittersweet for decorating the long farm table. I imagine her looking over her shoulder and hurrying back to the house when her arms were loaded with branches of orange berries. She never heard the crying, and I am sure she was just as glad. Sometimes it is a burden to see or hear through the mists between the worlds.

My grandmother would say, "I didn't sleep a wink last night. I heard that baby just crying and crying." My grandmother's dozen children were all grown by the time I heard her say those words, but she still felt the tug in her breast and the anxious need to gather up and cuddle. So she couldn't rest on the clear nights when that baby was beyond human comfort.

The old folks remembered the rotting logs of a cabin and stones from a chimney up Fox's Hollow, but by the time I was a child, even those were gone. No one could remember the names of the fierce-eyed man and the sad woman who had lived there. And no one ever knew the name of the baby whose fragile bones were found under the floorboards after the old man and woman died.

I am relieved these October sounds in Blackberry Cove are only a light wind in brittle leaves, water over stones in the run, and small creatures stirring the grass.

Tansy bounds up the steps and bumps me with her nose. She is still vibrant from some secret adventure, and her long hair is matted with cockleburrs. Dogs bring us right down to earth with their no-nonsense, here-and-now view of things. She will be a good companion this afternoon while I dig out the burdock and dandelion roots. She will nose around the groundhog hole while I fill a basket with windfalls from the old apple tree on our way up Timbrook's road to look for the last nettles. They are the sole spot of bright green as I gather the seeds into my sack with a gloved hand.

It will be relaxing for both of us tonight when she curls up beside me by the fire as I methodically untangle her cockleburrs. Halloween is still officially a week away, but I will remember the grandmothers' advice to burn up our useless chaff in October's fire and see events to come revealed in those Halloween flames.

Plantain

Rings of plantain (*Plantago major*) grow merrily around the huge stones that were once the foundation of a settler's cabin in Blackberry Cove.

Tons of plantain plants are pulled out of gardens and eradicated from our lawns every year. The fat oval leaves, tough fingers of pale yellow roots, and stalks of modest purple-green flowers are rarely recognized as a cherished medicinal herb with a long, noble history.

It came over with the grannies as a cultivated herb garden treasure. Soon our Appalachian birds discovered what Old World birds had always known—the tiny plantain seeds are nutritious and delicious. Before long, sunny places within bird-flight distance of settlements began to sprout with plantain. Native Americans called it "white man's foot" because they understood its origins and knew Europeans were in the area. They learned from the grandmothers that plantain was a medicinal herb useful in healing wounds and soon discovered it was good in treating snakebites as well. They gave it another of our folk-names, snakeweed.

In Scotland it is called Slan-lus, which means "plant of healing" in some local dialects. The Anglo-Saxons called it waybread and recognized it as one of their nine sacred herbs. The Appalachian grandmothers know a special salve that includes plantain will protect you from "flying venom."

Flying Venom Salve

Light a candle and say a prayer of protection before you combine the herbs and mix up the ingredients. Take a handful each of maythe (chamomile) and waybread (plantain), one-half an eggshell of honey, and three half eggshells of new butter. Work it with your hands into a salve. Melt it and strain it three times.

Plantain is an ingredient in many old ointments that also include comfrey, dock, and houseleeks, among various other herbs and flowers. A plain plantain salve is used by the grandmothers to soothe "all manner of spreading sores, tetters, ring-worm, and shingles."

Plantain Tea

Plantain tea is given by the grandmothers to ease diarrhea. They use it to strengthen the liver, to stop vomiting, and to drop into ears to ease the pain. When mixed with lemon juice, it is used as a diuretic.

Pour a pint of boiling water over a handful of fresh plantain leaves. Steep twenty minutes. Strain and cool. Take a quarter cup several times a day.

Plantain Seed Syrup

Country grandmothers recommend this for children with "thrush."

Boil a pint and a half of springwater down to a pint with an ounce of dried or fresh plantain seeds. Add a cup of honey or sugar. Cool and give one tablespoon, two or three times a day.

Fresh plantain leaves are an immediate country remedy for insect bites and cuts that occur out in the field. Just gather a few leaves, crush them up a little, and apply to the wound as an instant poultice.

Next time you look on that plantain with disdain—remember its virtues too. It was among the earliest plants recorded as growing in the first grandmothers' New World gardens. Maybe it cured a little homesickness, too!

Nettles

There is a thick patch of nettles along the steep dirt road that winds down from Black-berry Cove to the river. They are *Urtica dioica*, the common or stinging nettle, and will raise fiery red welts on your skin if you brush against them. As children, my cousins and I skipped over them on our way down the bank to the wild white water of the run. And if we were feeling wild ourselves, we thought it was hilarious to jostle each other into the nettle patch.

Those nettle stings don't last long, but I remember their bite when I wear gloves to cut bundles in the spring for drying. The whole plant is covered with stinging fuzz. Each of these tiny hairs is a hollow spine with minuscule amounts of an acrid ammonia-like fluid at its base. When there is pressure on the hair, the venom is pushed up and out.

Dock is the country antidote for nettle stings. It usually grows nearby, and the prescription is to rub fresh dock leaves on the welts and say three times:

Nettle in, dock out.
Dock rub nettle out!

Another version is to chant slowly while rubbing on dock leaves:

Out nettle, in dock.
Dock will have a new dress.
Nettle will not.

Our nettle blooms from early summer to nearly frost with plain green flowers clustered close to the stems where the heart-shaped toothed leaves sprout. Each plant usually has only male or female flowers. The male flowers bend outward, scattering pollen on the wind, where the more clustered female flowers catch it in a little brush. The perennial plant also multiplies by creeping roots, so it has become an unappreciated common weed.

It is another plant brought from the Old World as a valued companion. One grandfather said, "I have eaten nettles and I have slept on nettle sheets. I have heard my grandmother say nettle cloth is stronger than linen."

The name "nettle" comes from the Anglo-Saxon *netel*. The word "net" is a form of *ne*, an ancient common verb that means "spin and sew." The fiber is similar to hemp and flax, which were introduced from southern Europe to replace nettle. In Scotland, as late as the seventeenth century, nettle fibers were commonly used in weaving household cloth and fishing nets.

Nettle has an old reputation in the mountains as a healthy vegetable or potherb. Cooking heat dissipates the sting. The young tops should be gathered in the spring when they are five or six inches high. Wear gloves! Wash them in running water and cook in just a little springwater with the lid on for about twenty minutes. Serve with salt, pepper, and butter. They are delicious with eggs and gravy.

The grandmothers say cut nettle bunches just before they flower on a dry sunny day as the moon is getting full. Gather in loose bunches and dry in a dark warm place. As soon as the leaves are crispy, strip them off the stems and store in an air-tight tin. Once dried, they won't sting. Don't gather nettles for cooking or medicine after Summer Solstice—they form harmful crystals in the leaves.

Nettle Tea

Pour a pint of boiling springwater over a handful of dried nettle leaves and steep for ten minutes. Strain. Honey may be added.

The grandmothers say this is good for colds and flu, for healing damaged tissue, as a laxative, and as a diuretic. Nursing mothers give more milk when they drink nettle tea, say the grandmothers, and it smoothes out the hormonal dips and peaks of women going through the Change. They recommend a daily cup of nettle tea as a general strengthening tonic for everyone.

We know nettle is rich in calcium, magnesium, chlorophyll, and trace minerals. It has a high content of iron, potassium, and the B vitamins (especially thiamine), as well as vitamin A, vitamin C, vitamin D, vitamin K, selenium, and protein. The grandmothers know it stabilizes blood sugar, relieves chronic headaches, reduces allergies, and restores flagging energy.

When used as a lotion, the grandmothers tell, the cooled infusion is an antiseptic wash for burns and cuts, insect bites, and fungus infections.

Fresh nettle leaves applied directly to a wound help stop bleeding. Nettle leaves rubbed on stiff arthritic joints, say the grandmothers, will heat and loosen them up. The "burn" from nettles is really an intense tingling that can sometimes be pleasantly warming.

One old mountain remedy for a lingering fever is to reverently thank a nettle plant for its healing and then pull it up while saying the name of the person to be cured and reciting the names of his or her parents, grandparents, and ancestors as far back as you know. I love this way of honoring the plant and acknowledging our intimate kinship on the spiral of life.

Nettles were once recognized as good fodder for livestock. When they are growing, no animals will touch them, but when they are cut and dried, they are relished by cattle in particular. The grandmothers give dried nettle hay to their favorite milk cows to produce more and sweeter milk. Dried and powdered nettles in chicken feed increase egg production and make healthy birds. Pigs do well on boiled nettles, and gypsies mix nettle seed with oats for sleek, shiny horses.

Fresh nettles boiled with salt will curdle milk for cheese-making, and the same mixture rubbed on wooden barrels will make them waterproof. A strong decoction of nettle leaves will produce a beautiful green dye for wool.

I gather nettle seeds in early October when the time is just right. If I wait too long, the tiny seeds fall to the ground, so I keep a careful watch and shake the stalks into a brown paper bag when the seeds mature.

Nettle Seed Wine

This is good for fevers, flu, bronchitis, pneumonia, and whooping cough, say the grandmothers.

Soak a tablespoon of fresh or dried nettle seeds overnight in a glass of red wine. Warm it up, sweeten with honey or sugar, and sip all day.

Some grandmothers recommend a daily dose of a quarter teaspoon of dried nettle seed for thyroid problems. They also say nettle seeds stir up lust!

Burdock

Since our Shetland sheepdog gathers plenty of brown burdock sticker burrs in her tail every October, I rarely have to collect them myself. I just sit on the cabin floor in the evenings and help her untangle them. She gets to keep the soggy ones, and I make a pile of the dry intact ones. I will crumble the outer covering off with my fingers and separate out the little seeds from the downy fuzz around them.

The grandmothers say burdock seed tea is a powerful diuretic and soothing to the whole urinary system. The cooled infusion is also used as a skin lotion—for adolescents in particular.

Burdock Seed Tea

It only takes twenty-five or thirty dried seeds steeped in a cup of boiling springwater for ten minutes to make this tea.

Big coarse burdock (*Arctium lappa*) grows in the lower cove where the soil is rich and deep. The first year it produces those great arching leaves with reddish veins. It looks sort of like garden rhubarb. Only in the second year does it send up a flower stalk. That stalk grows from ankle high to shoulder tall in just a few days, and then blooms with little purple thistle-like flowers above those fat green stickle burrs.

The Appalachian grandmothers say it is these great wavy-edged first-year leaves that should be gathered fresh to wrap around skin abrasions, bruises, swollen joints, boils, burns, and just about any other skin irritation. They are a cooling healing poultice.

Plants that have many folk-names are usually beloved. Burdock may be cherished by the wise grandmothers, but it is shunned by shepherds and just about everyone else. Some of its other names are love leaves, beggar's buttons, cockle buttons, cockle-burs, thorny burr, stickers, sticktights, burrseed, harebur, cuckoo button, cloth burr, fox's clote, harelock, turkey burr, bat weed, and wooly dock.

The grandmothers say we should take cool bitter burdock leaf tea to lower a temperature and dampen a fiery temper. Taken hot, they say, with a little salt, it soothes indigestion caused by emotional distress and helps stop a lingering cough.

Burdock Leaf Tea

Gather one fresh burdock leaf and tear it into several pieces. Pour a pint of boiling spring-water over it and steep for several hours. Don't sweeten it. It has a nasty taste!

It is the burdock root, though, that the grandmothers love most of all. These sunny October days after the first frost and near a dark moon are perfect, they say, for digging burdock roots. You will need a sturdy spade and fork. Spade around the plant, starting and ending in the north. Then loosen the soil with your fork. That brown root will be deep! When it is pulled free, several of the lateral roots will probably break off, but that is good because a whole new burdock plant will grow from it next year.

If the root comes out too easily, it may be from a second-year plant in which the strength has already gone out of the root and into the seeds. That root will be worthless.

Scrub the root well in running water and use fresh if you can. If you must, dry it slowly in a warm place like a pilot-lit oven or the top of the refrigerator. The outside will be dark brown, but the inside of the burdock root will be white. Store whole and cut into inch-long pieces as you use it.

Burdock Root Tincture

At the dark of the moon fill a quart jar with chopped fresh burdock root. Fill the jar to the top with moonshine or 100 proof vodka. Store away in a dark place until the second full moon comes around. Then it is ready to use. Leave the burdock root in the alcohol and just take out what you need.

The grandmothers say twenty or thirty drops a day in springwater is a good tonic for the liver, uterus, kidneys, and digestive tract.

We now know burdock root is rich in iron, calcium, vitamins C and A, and trace minerals.

Burdock Root Tea

Pour a pint of boiling water over a cup of freshly chopped roots or a half-cup of dried chopped roots. Steep ten minutes. Strain. The tea has a pleasant sweetness of its own, but you can add honey.

The grandmothers recommend taking a half-cup a day for weak lungs, uterus, stomach, kidneys, and liver, and to increase energy generally. Burdock root infusion cooled and used as a lotion, they say, soothes cold sores, rashes, hives, and fungus infections. Rinse your hair with it if you have chronic dandruff.

The mountain grandmothers agree burdock works best for people with patience. It is a slow and steady worker, reaching the deepest parts of ourselves where real transformation takes place.

Wild Apples

The ancient gnarled apple tree that greets us as we turn in the lane to Blackberry Cove has a mysterious pedigree. Just about the only botanical name we can safely give it is *Malus*, but we love it dearly. When the tree split almost in half one winter, we fretted. But it leafed out gloriously that spring despite its cracked and nearly hollow trunk, and even the fallen limbs bloomed. Now we savor the few wildlings the deer leave us in the fall and are grateful for every season Old Man Apple is green.

The Appalachian grandmothers call the oldest tree in the apple orchard the Apple Tree Man and pay it great reverence. Blackberry Cove's Old Man Apple must surely be King of the Apple Tree Men.

For several years after we came to the cove, we nibbled on little green apples in the summer and waited for them to grow fat, yellow, and sweet. When we thought they would be just ripe enough, we made a special trip to the cove. And they had disappeared! Only a few little misshapen ones were left. It was a great mystery. I said to my father one day, "Do all those apples fall at one time, and do the deer eat them in one big midnight feast?"

"I don't think so," he said. "Years ago Dad told Uncle Tom he could have the apples off that tree."

So we honored that old pledge. Then one year my father's uncle Tom didn't come with his children to collect his apples, and we heard he had crossed to where the magical apple trees of Avalon always bear both blossoms and fruit. Now we call them Uncle Tom's apples and only share them with the deer, rabbits, raccoons, and groundhogs.

Apples of every kind have been a staple in cool weather areas of the world since long before recorded history. They are nutritious (full of vitamin C, among others), store well all year, and can be made into all sorts of alcoholic ciders and ales. Even today every family has a favorite apple recipe—as American as apple pie.

These eastern foothills of the Appalachians are apple country. Grandfather Osa had a wide commercial orchard right on top of the mountain where you could see for miles all around. My mother says her schoolday "dinners" were almost always dark rich apple butter on crusty homemade bread. Soggy by noontime. And when I was born just after World War II, my young parents were living in the big white farmhouse with my grandparents. Since they didn't even have a cradle, Grandfather Osa offered to put me up temporarily in one of his sturdy wooden apple boxes.

There are apple harvest fairs in every little village and apple-butter making at every country church. The big town of Winchester has a grand Apple Blossom Festival every year in May and crowns a beautiful Apple Blossom Queen and her court of Princesses.

But up in the hills the grandmothers know rotten apples rubbed on an obstinate sty will soothe it, and a rotten apple stuck on a sore toe will ease the pain. They say if a child has the chicken pox, set a ripe apple in the child's room. As the apple begins to get spots, the spots on the child will fade.

If the sun shines through the bare apple branches on Old Christmas Day (January 6) it foretells a grand apple crop next summer. That is also the night, instruct the grandmothers, to go Apple Howling to insure abundant apples in the coming season. Men go out to the orchard and pass the cider jar around the trees with mighty shouts, howls, and even gun blasts into the air. The old song is:

Here's to thee
Old Apple Tree!
Whenst thou mayst blow
And whenst thou mayst bear
Apples enow:
Hats full!
Caps full!
Bushels, bushels, sacks full
And my pockets full too!
Huzza! Huzza!

Some mountain grandmothers actually call Halloween "Snap-Apple Night" and say women can tell if their mates are true by putting apple seeds in the fire that night and saying:

If you love me, pop and fly.
If you hate me, lay and die.

And almost every country girl has peeled an apple in one long paring, thrown it back over her left shoulder, and turned around clockwise to see the letter it formed—the initial of her husband-to-be. Boys flip an apple seed up in the air and say:

North, south, east, west,
Tell me where my girl does rest.

If an apple blossom appears on the tree at the same time as fruit in the fall, whisper some grandmothers, it foretells that a member of the family will cross to the mystical Isle of Apples before spring.

Lazy Larry is the guardian spirit of apple orchards, tell other grandmothers. He sometimes appears as a colt to chase away thieves. If the rascals steal any apples, Lazy Larry casts a spell on them:

Cramps, crooking and lose their footing.

Sauces and pies and butters and dumplings are best left to those coddled domestic apples. I love the tart and twisted wildlings right from our old tree. Henry Thoreau said it best:

To appreciate the wild and sharp flavor of these October fruits, it is necessary that you be breathing the sharp October or November air. The out-door air and exercise which the walker gets give a different tone to his palate and he craves a fruit which the sedentary would call harsh and crabbed. They must be eaten in the fields, when your system is all aglow with exercise, when the frosty weather nips your fingers, the wind rattles the bare boughs and rustles the few remaining leaves, and the jay is heard screaming around. What is sour in the house a bracing walk makes sweet.

November

It is pure Indian Summer when I drive down into Blackberry Cove. The air is momentarily still, and persimmons hanging from the nearly leafless little tree at the end of the lane are brilliant orange in the warm sun. They are already softened and sweetened by the hard frosts of November, just right for gathering now.

Black walnuts litter the clearing around the cabin, still encased in their hard green outer covering. After a snow or two those pungent citrus-fragranced rinds will turn black and be easier to scrape away from the nut, but I make a silent note to gather them soon. One quick gray squirrel is already racing up and down tree trunks amassing her winter store. Children here in the Appalachians are told that squirrels are messengers between the birds in treetops and the little creatures like worms and grubs who burrow into the soil. There must be lots of news on this day!

Even these warm-blooded squirrels will soon settle in for the winter rest, emerging only briefly in midday, remembering their hidden treasures. Seeds and eggs are nestled in by now, and frogs and toads and turtles have expertly buried themselves for sleeping.

Tansy, however, is frisking all over the clearing this afternoon. She barks up the tree at the squirrel, then is up to the spring, back down, unable to keep still. Mountain wisdom says a boisterous dog foretells stormy weather.

We both saw a sleek black dog lope across the road on our way in. Tansy's ears stood up and she watched intently for as long as we could see it disappear in the brush. I instinctively made a cross in the air above the steering wheel, as my mother and aunts always do when a black animal (especially a cat) crosses in front. Not a real "sign of the cross," mind you! These women are staunch Calvinists! Their sign and mine is a quick little X at arm's length. The grandmothers recite this short charm, too. "Black dog, Black dog, go on your way. Leave good luck with me, and bless this day."

In the highlands, huge black dog spirits are thought to roam the countryside. Here is one of the grandmother stories.

Once upon a time on the darkest night a man set out through the woods to visit his old and desperately sick mother in her cabin. It was a wild night. The wind moaned and whistled. Out of nowhere appeared a little old lady with a cheery smile. "It is a dangerous night," she said. "My dog will walk with you. But don't look back at it and keep walking until you get to your old mother's house."

The man thanked her and wondered how she knew where he was going. He felt better, though, with the sound of the dog pad-pad-padding along behind him.

When he got to his old mother's cabin and opened the door, she screamed from her bed, "What is that?" When he turned around the man saw the biggest black dog with the biggest yellow eyes shining out.

"Don't worry mother, he's a good dog," said the man, and the dog settled down in front of the door, wagging his tail.

In the morning the man's mother was completely well again, and the big dog was nowhere to be seen.

This November sunset comes quickly, its long slanting light touching the leafless hills for one moment of redness before they turn a deep chilled purple.

I am glad to be tucked inside the cabin myself when the wind picks up in the darkness outside. At first it swirls gently around the cabin, the last leaves skittering over the roof and against the glass. But by midnight it is roaring down the mountain. Wet November winds in these Appalachians come in bone-chilling blasts from Canada, scattering even the memories of summer and leaving only sear stalks and bare tree branches.

I catch a comforting glimpse of my Grandmother LuLu Catherine's face in the woodstove flames, and I remember how mountain women knew the power and magic of wind.

"One afternoon in the fall of the year," Lulu Catherine said, "I was hanging up wash on the long line across the ditch when there come a wind. I heard it roaring and I thought, it is going to rain. But there wasn't a cloud in the sky and not a branch was blowing. My clothes were hanging straight down. It was just that sound of wind.

"I went back in the house and it wasn't a minute or two before the woman up the road came running with her baby in her arms. The poor little thing was just dead, already blue. There was nothing we could do, and I know that wind was taking her sweet soul away," my grandmother would repeat in the same sad and quiet voice.

The great-great-grandmothers from across the sea not only knew the mystery of wind, they knew how to use it, call it up at will, and disperse it with their own breath. But we have long forgotten the ways. Now we respect these changes wrought by wind, feel its power in our blood, and know only fragments of our heritage in such passed-down ditties as "When the wind is in the east, 'Tis neither good for man nor beast."

After a restless night I awaken early in the gray bone-chilling cabin where every coal in the stove has burned down to a damp pile of ashes. Cold rain pelts the windows. I know it will be a miserable day to gather nuts or persimmons, so I brew up a cup of strong black tea and pack up as quickly as I can. Even Tansy has given up chewing on the big burdock tangle in her tail and is waiting by the door. We both are looking forward to a nice hot breakfast at the truckstop on the way back to town.

Pokeweed

Spring poke-sallet greens are a tasty delicacy in the Appalachians, but the grandmothers wait until early November and well after frost to gather poke roots and berries.

Poke (*Phytolacca americana*) grows as tall as a small tree at the edges of the upper meadow in Blackberry Cove. The big fleshy perennial looks nearly tropical and out of place on our mountain. By summer the leaves are huge, and by late fall big clusters of black-purple berries hang heavily. Those green leaves and stems are poisonous, and the berry flesh is eaten safely only by the birds.

But the mountain grandmothers use that purple berry juice as a rub for skin eruptions. They dig the roots to dry and crush them into springwater for a poultice applied to the soles and palms of a feverish person. Native Americans taught them how to use the dried powdered poke roots to treat skin cancers when better methods weren't available.

Some other folk-names are American nightshade, cancer root, cokum, crow berry, inkberry, pigeon berry, red-ink plant, red wood, scoke, Virginia poke, and devil's club.

The berry juice makes a nearly permanent reddish purple ink or stain—which birds love to drop on our cars, hanging laundry, and freshly painted fences.

One country grandmother says she uses one or two dried poke berries a day for easing joint pains. Swallow the dried berries whole without crushing the seed, and they aren't toxic, she says. The seeds pass right on out.

I enjoy the beauty of poke most in the fall when the leaves fade and those jeweled clusters of berries take center stage. I think of poke-bonneted grandmothers cutting the new shoots for greens, digging the healing roots, and gathering the beautiful berries. I think of the edge of fear in pokeweed's poisonous leaves and enticing fruit. It is the quintessential wild Appalachian herb.

Persimmon

There is a whole persimmon (*Diospyros virginiana*) grove along the road over the mountain by old Number Six Schoolhouse, but in Blackberry Cove we have just one tree. It stands alone in the meadow across the lane from the apple tree.

We nearly always miss the small creamy yellow flowers in late spring and hardly notice the tree at all in summer and early fall. But on certain dark gray November days, the little frosted-orange persimmons stand out like Christmas lights on the crooked black branches.

It is a windy day after several hard frosts when it's time to shake down the persimmons. By now their dark pumpkin-colored skin is wrinkled, and the light inside is soft and luscious. There are six or eight flat seeds inside that rich fruit, which tastes like sweet ripe plums or figs with a tangy hint of wildness. It is good luck to recite the old mountain ditty as you shake the tree:

> *Possum up the simmon tree.*
> *Raccoon on the ground.*
> *Raccoon says, "You son of a _____!*
> *Shake them simmons down."*

Sometimes by the time we get there, the birds, raccoons, and possums have just about polished off the sweet little fruit, and we get just one or two to eat right away.

Even after the first few frosty nights when the fruit is firm and orange, it makes you pucker. Captain John Smith of Jamestown wrote, "it will draw a man's mouth awrie with much torment." I don't think there is an Appalachian child who hasn't been suckered by the older kids into trying an unripe persimmon. It is a mountain rite of passage.

If you are lucky to get a basketful of ripe persimmons, they are good to use right away or can be nicely frozen. Don't wash them, just pick off the dried flower sepals that cling to their ends and put them in a freezer bag.

Here is one grandmother's fall recipe:

Persimmon Bread

1 cup persimmon pulp, fresh or frozen and thawed
  (with skins but without seeds)
2 eggs
1 cup sugar
2 cups flour sifted with 3 tablespoons baking powder and a pinch of salt
1/2 cup of vegetable oil
1 cup chopped pecans

Beat together the persimmon, eggs, and sugar until creamy. Stir in flour mixture, oil, and pecans. Spread in a loaf pan and bake at 325°F for an hour.

Persimmons have more vitamin C than oranges and lots of potassium and iron. They are a source of quick energy with their extremely high content of natural sugar.

The Native Americans who taught the grandmothers about persimmons called it "pasimen." Some other English names are date plum, possumwood, seeded plum, simmon, and plum.

Those grandmothers learned to make an infusion of green fruit to ease diarrhea. That same bitter tea soothes a sore throat. The Indian grandmothers taught them how to dry and powder persimmon seed for mixing with rainwater to treat kidney stones. Persimmon roots gathered in the fall and boiled up in springwater, they learned, make a remedy for dysentery. The grandmothers were taught to gather pieces of the broken scaly bark squares in the spring to boil up in a decoction to cool and wash the sore mouths of nursing babies.

And they learned from their Indian neighbors to honor and thank the persimmon tree and the possums who share it.

Black Walnut

We have one black walnut (*Juglans nigra*) tree growing within hugging distance of the cabin deck. It is tall and spare—the last tree to leaf out in the spring and the first to shed yellow leaves in the earliest fall. It gives practically no shade at all, but we love the sound of those crisp oval leaves rattling in the breeze and the roughness of its dark ribbed trunk.

The truly great and grand black walnuts grow in the rich river-bottom soil around my father's homeplace down the road. There is a whole grove of them, each rising more than one hundred feet tall.

In November the yard is thick with those nubby round green hulls. Later they will turn black and crumble away to give up the hard crinkly black walnuts with their precious kernels.

My uncle Arlie often had dark-stained hands this time of year from when he hulled black walnuts. His favorite way of separating the nuts from the fleshy black hulls was to pour a bushel of them on the ground under his huge tractor tires and run back and forth over them.

One year my father spent weeks cracking the tough black walnuts with my grandfather's old iron contraption made especially for the task. He painstakingly picked out that rich delicious nut meat. I volunteered to make a wonderful black walnut pound cake for him. I made that cake, which sagged in the middle—barely rising more than an inch. It was a disaster! I'll never get another black walnut from him again.

Our splendid black walnuts on these western slopes of the Shenandoah Valley are richly flavorful with an underlying subtlety of wild mushrooms and the aroma of deep black soil.

Black Walnut Butter

1/2 cup of finely chopped black walnuts
1/2 cup of butter at room temperature
1/4 teaspoon of brown sugar
a tiny pinch of nutmeg

Cream together. This is wonderful on toast for breakfast.

Black Walnut Pie

1 cup sugar
1 cup dark corn syrup
2 tablespoons of butter
3 eggs
1 tablespoon of pure vanilla extract
1 cup of black walnuts, chopped coarsely
1 single unbaked pastry crust

Boil sugar and syrup slowly until the mixture begins to thicken. Add the butter and vanilla. Beat eggs in a separate bowl. Pour mixture slowly into the eggs, beating all the while. Sprinkle the black walnuts over the bottom of the pastry shell and pour the syrup mixture over them. Bake at 425°F for ten minutes. Reduce heat to 350°F and bake for forty-five minutes longer. Serve cold with fresh thick cream.

This part of West Virginia and over the hills in Virginia is so lush with native black walnut trees that the earliest cabinetmakers here used the beautifully grained walnut wood not only for the showy fronts of furniture, but also for the unseen backs and drawer bottoms that are usually pine. In our Harpers Ferry dining room stands a tall graceful cupboard made for a member of my father's family in the early nineteenth century. Every inch of its wood is black walnut.

The early Appalachian grandmothers recognized the native black walnut as a close cousin to their great European walnut trees. Some other names for it are welsh nut, Jupiter's nuts, and, from the German grandmothers, nutzbaum.

The Italian grandmothers knew the secrets of *noci* (walnuts), too. My husband's Italian grandparents delighted in little delicacies of two walnut halves with a fig between. Then one day I came across these lines from a sixteenth-century herbal:

Dry walnuts taken with a fig withstand poison, prevent and preserve the body from the infection of plague, and being plentifully eaten they drive worms forth of the belly.

Mountain grandmothers make a poultice of onions, black walnuts, salt, and honey to treat carbuncles. They boil black walnut meats with sugar to comfort the stomach and expel poison. They know the oil pressed from black walnuts makes hands and faces smooth and takes away black and blue marks.

The new leaves and first buds steeped in boiling springwater make a tea to help stop "loose bowels," they say. The same cooled tea used as a lotion to bathe the body will help "procure sweat." And a decoction of the green hulls with their tangy citrus-like smell and flavor will help stay diarrhea.

The grandmothers know it is the worst of luck when a black walnut tree falls—whatever the reason.

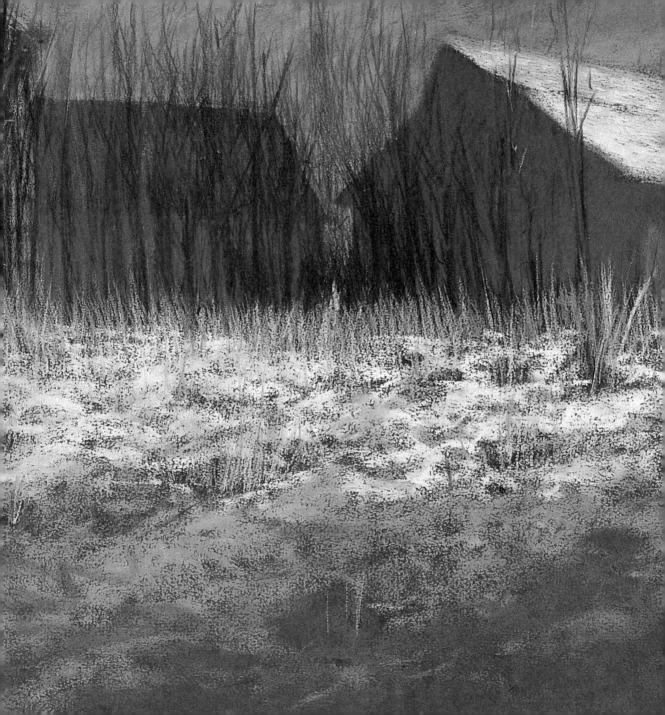

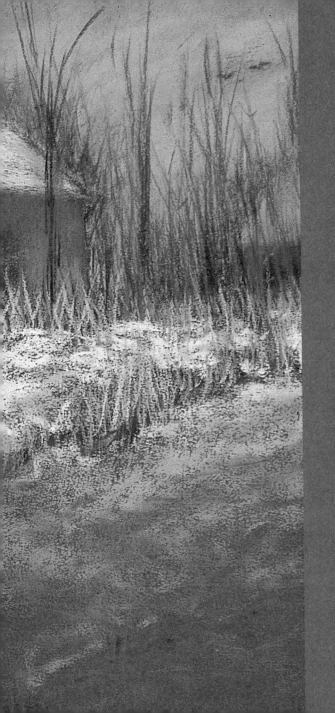

Winter

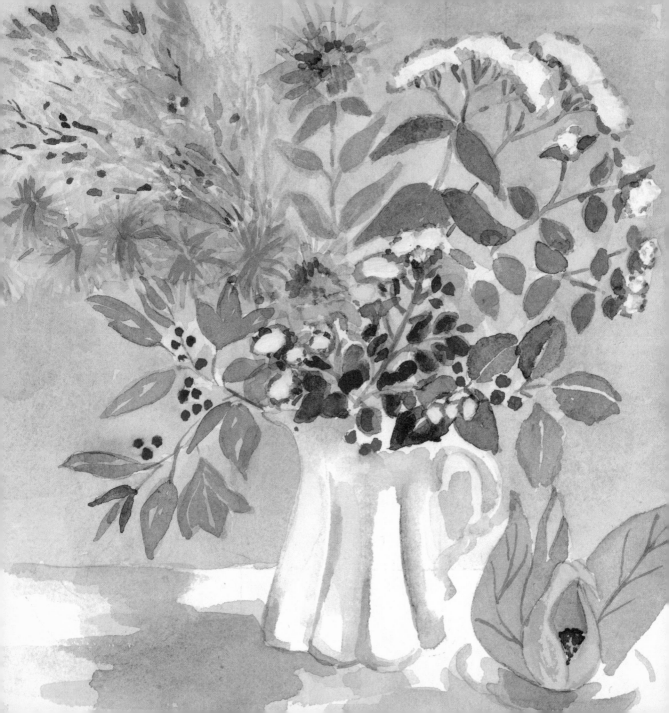

December

This brief December dusk has already slipped into darkness as I drive the winding road through Mill Creek Valley. Narrow but paved, it hugs the western side of this ribbon of a valley, following the ridges in and out as they flatten into fields. You can nearly step from the porches of the old houses right onto the macadam. I think about how the valley has changed only slightly since I first brought my husband down this road over thirty years ago, chattering to him.

"My uncle Floyd lives in that house. My grandmother's people, the Davys and the McDonalds, are from up that lane. See that long house right on the road? My great-grandmother Harriet lived there as a little girl during the Civil War. Her mother had died, so she lived with her oldest sister, the innkeeper's wife. In the attic they hid Confederate soldiers caught behind Union lines when the lines shifted. The men in the family had to take the oath of Allegiance to the Union, but the women didn't, so they fed and cared for those boys in butternut until they could escape."

"Great-aunt Effie lives in that white house, and Uncle Ernie keeps this general store. Grandma says you can still dig out miniballs from that bank over there where the Yankees shot target."

1. Watercress; 2. Sassafras; 3. Witch Hazel; 4. Red Cedar;
5. Mountain Mint; 6. Boneset; 7. Chickweed; 8. Wintergreen;
9. Skunk Cabbage

By the time we had driven up the valley to "the head of the lane," where the dirt road turns off to both of my grandparents' farms, his New York City ears were ringing with my entire genealogy. I didn't tell him some of the weirder stories until after we were married and he couldn't be scared off.

I smile to myself in the dark this evening as I think about what a good sport he has been all these years. What a puzzlement this wild Appalachian family must have been for him. Like a good New Yorker, he always shrugged and accepted. Now I think these mountains have cast their spell over him too, as he has felt their seasons circle for more than half of his own life.

The jeep slows down to turn the sharp curve where an ancient and deserted log house crumbles beside the road, and I remember Aunt Maggie's story. She wasn't really my aunt by blood, but she was beloved as "Aunt Maggie" by everyone in the valley when she died a few years ago at 101. The oldest of a big family and never married, she looked after her siblings and parents and then traveled to other families when they needed extra help with a new baby or a bad sickness.

"One night," she told, "we were coming home from a Christmas program at Mt. Olive Church. Mother and Dad sat up front on the wagon, and because it was frosty cold, we kids were bundled up in the back. You know that long straight in the road right as you come out of Mt. Olive? Well, it was along there that I heard Mother say there was a woman walking alone in the road up ahead. Then we all looked and saw her. Mother wondered to Dad who she might be, and said we would give her a lift on this bitter night. Just as we got up beside her at the turn in the road by that log house, she disappeared. We all called out, thinking maybe she fell or something, but she had just disappeared into thin air."

I shiver as I round the curve tonight, wondering myself about the mysterious woman and considering how easily country people accept the unexplained in the dark of the night.

We are just a few days from the longest night of the year, the Winter Solstice. In the yearly cycle of sunlight, we now pay the balance due on those long warm summer days.

I shut the jeep lights in Blackberry Cove and sit for a moment to let my eyes get accustomed to the dark. The bright crescent of a waning moon rides over the ridge, and the darkness thins around me. The cove glows with an incandescent shimmer.

Tansy and I sit outside for a while as the moon rides high over this cold and brittle night of magic, a night as long as a day in June, a star night as well as a moon night. The Dipper looks within easy reach, and the Milky Way arches over the cove like star-dust from a good witch's wand. I stay out until my nose is nearly frozen, and even then I am reluctant to leave this long, sweet darkness.

The mountain grandmothers sometimes called the Milky Way "Cow's Lane" be-cause whoever gave a cow to help the poor would be led after death by that same cow over the Milky Way and safely into Paradise. Cows are holy beasts.

My own grandmother loved her cows dearly. She always had a pair of Guernseys that she milked twice a day in the sturdy little barn my grandfather had built. She kept her big family supplied with fresh milk most of the year and even sometimes sold cream and butter for extra cash.

Some of my earliest memories are of those wonderful barn smells of warm milk, hay, and sweet cow's breath. Barn cats of every color made a crescent behind Grand-mother's milking stool, waiting patiently until she filled upturned old hubcaps with milk from her bucket. Sometimes, most fascinating of all, she turned around without missing a beat and squirted milk directly from the teat into a hubcap.

Nearly every spring Grandmother would be excited about a new little fawn-colored calf. If it were a male or her milk cows were still hardy, my uncle would take it to mar-ket in the summer. If the calf was a particularly likely heifer, she would become an honored milk cow.

Cows are said by mountain people to live in close spiritual harmony with their owners, sharing happiness and sorrow. At midnight on Winter Solstice they talk to one another, predicting the fate of their families and the community for the coming year.

The grandmothers whisper stories about little fairy cows, no bigger than a small dog, who could sometimes be seen grazing with regular cows. They would protect them and give warnings of danger. Sometimes the fairy cow would grow huge and fat and give abundant milk in lean times. If the family became too greedy, though, the fairy cow would disappear.

The ancient Celtic Earth Goddess would often appear as a white cow in two guises. One was as nourisher and protector and the other as mean and cranky, banishing her young from the herd. The grandmothers say this is to teach children otherwise stunted in their development to grow up and look out for themselves.

The grandmothers say cows have such sweet breath because a cow saw the baby Jesus shivering in the manger at midnight and warmed him with her breath. Now a cow's breath is healing and wholesome, and she carries her young nine months in harmony with our own mothers.

The most revered cow of all, though, is the dun cow. Dun means brown, so I think of my grandmother's beautiful Guernseys, but dun is also a Celtic word that means royal. I also think of her majestic cows.

In just a few days the sunlight will begin to lengthen. Today we can predict just when and by how much, but it is still only faith. We know it has happened every year before, and we believe the light and warmth will return again this year. But tonight it doesn't seem so strange that our ancestors sang and celebrated and drummed the rhythms of pulses and cycles of the year to keep the great wheel turning, bringing back the light.

Almost every culture in every part of the world has a midwinter celebration of light to entice the sun. Beneath our own Christmas rituals of plastic Santas, we still find joy in the eternal green of holly and pine, the sparkle of candles, the excitement of mistletoe, and the delight in a newborn child bringing light.

Daylight comes over the mountain in blue spreading to rose. It is a cold light this morning, and I am reluctant to move from my warmth under three quilts. There is a fire to be made and tea to be brewed before I will be warm enough to set out on my quest for greens to decorate the house in Harpers Ferry.

I want to cut a basket of small twigs from sassafras and witch hazel trees on my way up the mountain, and at midday I want to walk the ridge above the cabin. At this time of year the view from there is of endless mountains stretching westward.

So it is early afternoon when we begin to pack up. Cloud cover has turned the sky a dull white, and on this short December day the light is already dimming when the jeep bumps onto the paved road.

Sassafras

Between the cabin and the spring are several young sassafras (*Sassafras albidum*) trees with their unusual mitten leaves. Some are three-lobed and some are single ovals or fan-shaped like the leaves on older trees, but we still call them mitten trees and look for a matched pair of mittens.

Sassafras has had some aspersions cast on its character in recent years. Scientists have told us sassafras is carcinogenic. The grandmothers agree it is a powerful herb, so if we are greedy and misuse its goodness, it can indeed be harmful. But, they maintain, one hearty cup of pink sassafras root tea every spring will charge up your metabolism and thin your winter-sluggish blood.

The oldest Appalachian grandmothers say we should find a spot plentiful with sassafras seedlings. Then after a hard frost in December, near the dark of the moon, tell the whole grove that you appreciate their strength and beauty and need their good medicine. Pull up one entire small seedling, cut off the whole top, and save the

roots. Wash them well in running water, cut in three-inch lengths, dry slowly in a
warm oven, and store away until spring.

In early spring place five pieces of root in a pot with a quart of cold springwater.
Bring to a boil and simmer gently for fifteen minutes. The water will turn a rosy color.
Sweeten with sugar or honey. Take no more than a cup a day for several days.

Save the roots, dry them again, and reuse them over and over until the decoction
no longer turns pink or has that distinctive sassafras aroma.

Some mountain grandmothers use only root bark from mature trees. Some
Louisiana grandmothers gather the new leaves, dry them, and rub them into filé
powder (a mixture of dry spices) to flavor their rich gumbos.

The first Native American grandmothers taught us how to use sassafras to ease
menstrual cramps and the afterpains of childbirth. They rubbed sassafras juice on
sore joints and rubbed sassafras leaves on sore teeth and gums.

Sassafras is one of the loveliest and most loved of our small native trees. Tip your
hat to her!

Witch Hazel

On the northern bank, just as the road to Blackberry Cove goes through a deep gap,
grows a whole stand of little witch hazel trees (*Hamamelis virginiana*). I first noticed
them years ago when they blossomed with their crinkly hanging stars of the brightest
yellow during cold December when everything around them was brown and gray.

They have the peculiar habit of blooming after their leaves have fallen, just at the
edge of deep winter. Witch hazel is the most brazen gambler in the forest since it can
be pollinated only by those last hardy insects who come alive on short sunny December afternoons.

Those very witch hazel's forebears must have been there when my grandfather,
his horse, and his fancy new "courting buggy" went over the bank right below them.

The family says he was coming home alone from seeing my grandmother on the blackest, iciest night when his horse lost its footing and over the bank they tumbled. No one was hurt—the witch hazels witnessed it all.

Hanging on our wall at home is a faded, sun-softened photograph of solemn young Grandfather Osa with Grandmother Lulu Catherine, all dressed up and sitting side by side in a perky little buggy. Must have been before the fall!

Witch hazel is the most magical of Appalachian trees. According to the grandmothers, a three-pronged witch hazel stick cut in the rain during the waning moon of February makes the most powerful divining rod of all for water dowsers.

Woodland Indians showed the early grandmothers how to gather the round witch hazel leaves in summer, the bark in fall, and the beautiful crooked twigs in early spring.

Freshly peeled bark, say the grandmothers, can be laid directly on skin inflammations to speed healing. Chewed bark sweetens the breath and soothes mouth sores.

Fresh or dried witch hazel twigs steeped in a bathtub full of hot water makes a wonderful and fragrant bath for easing sore muscles and hemorrhoids.

Even today every drugstore carries bottles of witch hazel lotion. Use it for rubbing on bruises or sprains, as an antiseptic for small cuts, and as shaving lotion. The grandmothers say runners should rub witch hazel lotion on their legs to keep limber. It is easy, they say, to make your own lotion.

Witch Hazel Lotion

Fill a quart jar as full as possible with any combination of fresh witch hazel leaves, twigs, and/or bark. Then pour in rubbing alcohol to the top of the jar. Cover and set in a dark place from one full moon to the next. When it is ready to use, you can strain it out into smaller bottles or just use it directly from the jar. Leave the witch hazel plant material in the jar!

Red Cedar

Each December we cut a full and fragrant red cedar tree to put in the place of honor by the tall front window in Harpers Ferry. We decorate it with as many tiny lights as the delicate branches can hold and suspend the lightest of ornaments from their tips.

The red cedar is the Christmas tree of my childhood. It is the traditional tree in these hills and valleys, where it was cut from the wild and brought inside long before commercial tree farms appeared. Red cedars are so plentiful here that farmers are always glad to clear them from orchards and pastures.

They are really a species of native juniper as we can see in their botanical name, *Juniperus virginiana.* They are holy trees. Long before the first Appalachian grandmothers came from the Old World, they venerated the sacred juniper as the tree of sanctuary. Juniper's dense thickets of sharp needles make safe hiding places for small creatures, and the strong pungent odor of the red cedar juniper masks the scent of the hiding animal.

Once upon a time in the widest valley, furthest from the hills, a sweet-faced young mother decided to quietly pack up her new babe and set out before dawn for home. Her boy-of-a-husband and his family in the hip-roofed brick house frowned when she left her shoes by the door to run barefoot in the garden. They scorned her lilting mountain words and tsked-tsked when she suckled her newborn with her own rich milk. She longed to hear the wild winds around her mother's cabin and her father's loud laughter inside. So in the darkest of the night, she set out on foot for home.

When her husband and his brothers discovered her empty bed, they mounted swift black horses and rode out after her.

In the blue hour before sunrise she heard them coming. The red cedar junipers in the thicket around her opened their spiny branches and folded them around her, soft and downy inside, while the black horses thudded right past.

When they were gone and away, she gathered up her baby and made her way between the mountains, up to the warm cabin where her mother and father, brothers and sisters, and all the grandmothers welcomed her home.

We still decorate with our native junipers of sanctuary and sometimes plant them by our doors where black witches are compelled to count every needle before they can come inside. When they lose count (and they always do, say the grandmothers), they are bound to start over. Eventually those mean conjurers get discouraged and go away.

The grandmothers say we should burn the aromatic blue berry-like cones to keep away bad luck and thunderbolts. Smoke from the burning wood and needles was once recommended to keep away "all infection, corruption of the aire which bringeth the plague and such like contagious disease."

The mountain grandmothers boil the leaves and twigs in water to make a steam inhaled as treatment for bronchitis. They make a warm poultice of boiled berries to relieve rheumatism. A weak tea made from the leaves and twigs will help restore lost strength, they say.

Too many desperate and untrained countrywomen, whisper the grandmothers, have died from taking strong boiled-down juniper decoctions to induce abortion.

Be wary of the red cedar's sharp needles, they counsel, and respect her power. If we protect her goodness, she will protect ours.

January

January on the Blue Ridge is usually a time of crystalline purity. The only visible life around us is in the garden of frost flowers on our windowpanes each morning before the sun gathers them.

I rarely visit Blackberry Cove in January because the steep and twisting road would be impossible to climb if an unexpected storm came over the Allegheny Mountains. The cabin rests in my imagination, still and cold with only a crow flapping through the trees and the spring piling up ice sculptures down the run.

But this year the January thaw comes early, opening winter's door a crack, so I pack up a winter picnic and set off to Blackberry for the day. I am just going to check on the cabin. Mother Nature does her pruning this time of year, and she's not particular about where her branches fall. I'll make sure the roof is still strong and the lane is clear, but the real reason I go is for the simple joy of being outside again.

On this day the brief winter sun is almost warm by noon. A slick of mud on top of the frozen ground makes the gooey road as slippery as black ice, but the cabin is wintering safely.

My imaginary crow has turned into a pair of real ones, cawing raucously in the topmost branches of a scraggly old walnut tree. These huge black birds (*Corvus brachyrhynchos*), who mischievously raid gardens in early spring, are dark winter prophets of the Appalachian soul. Instinctively I give them my careful attention. The grandmothers said they carried secrets of life and death, foretelling wars and disasters. Our native crows must have recalled for them the great flapping ravens of Scotland, who could sometimes speak to them in their own language and sometimes let the wisest of them understand bird language. These old women said crows embodied earthbound human spirits, and if a crow were killed, the nearest baby would wail in sorrow. So I listen to these winter crows, but hear no ominous message today. I do smile, though, when I remember that crows can foretell lighter events, closer to home. One mountain ditty is, "If a crow cries right o'er her head, she's soon to lose her maidenhead."

The spring is bubbling out with only a rim of lacy ice along its path, and a few tiny leaves of watercress are still green in a lower pool. When I scratch down under the newest layer of fallen leaves on the south-facing slope of Owl Mountain, I find a handful of bronzed green mountain mint leaves at the base of a dead stalk. They are wonderfully fragrant.

This little treasure of chlorophyll makes me consider our foremothers' store of dried herbs in wooden boxes or hanging in smoky kitchens, ready for January's maladies. There must have been huge coltsfoot leaves and crinkly horehound for lingering coughs. Sage for sore throats, and boneset for flu and fever.

I heat water on the round old stove and draw up a chair to the last glows of the fire. It has a long heritage, this cup of tea to soothe and cure. I think the parts we've most forgotten are the incantations breathed over the pot. "Let my baby breathe easier." "Let this brew ease Grandpa's aching legs." The magic was most powerful when loving hands gathered and dried the herbs, heartfelt wishes (along with the honey) sweetened the broth, and warm fingers curled around the cup.

By four o'clock the sun leaves the cove with just a faint glow of orange light along the ridge, backlighting the braid of black tree branches. Mud is crunching underfoot. It is this rhythmic freeze and thaw of Appalachian winters that slowly breaks up the rocks themselves, and over millions of years has softened our mountains into their great round beauty.

As I drive back to town in the dark I'm grateful that January relented and give thanks for the respite. Now it's time to burrow in again to let winter thoughts form in their own good way. It is time for long dark nights filled with dreams of talking crows. It is time to pull out the heavy old books about the winter herbs and dig into their roots.

Watercress

The exquisite little watercress (*Nasturtium officinale*) that grows so abundantly even during January in the streams of our Appalachian foothills is in the Cruciferae (or mustard) family of plants. In fact the word "cress" is an old Anglo-Saxon word for mustard-like plant. Mountain people sometimes call it tang-tongue because of its biting taste, and its scientific name, *Nasturtium*, comes from the Latin "twisted nose," referring to the sharpness of watercress.

The stem grows horizontally submerged in springwater with small white roots wiggling in the stream current. Succulent, smooth, and vividly green pinnate leaves are one to six inches long with three to nine leaflets. In June tiny white flowers with four petals appear briefly before maturing into long slender seed pods.

Fishermen like to see watercress in a stream because they know it often means a good trout habitat for breeding and food. Be careful that you gather watercress from clean water, though, because unfortunately some of our streams are contaminated, and it will thrive there as well.

Watercress is not a native plant to North America. It found its way from Europe with the early settlers over the Blue Ridge, where it has naturalized in our mountain streams.

Our ancestors didn't know watercress was extremely rich in vitamin C, but they knew its pungent leaves were a good spring tonic. Ancient Romans prescribed watercress leaves to quiet deranged minds!

English herbalist John Gerard called it "Water Cresse" or "Water Parsenep," "fat and full of juice." He said boiled in wine or milk, it is good against scurvy. "Boiled in a broth with meat and eaten for 30 days at morning, noon and night it provokes urine and draws down stones. Also in young maidens it brings on their menses."

Watercress pottage (leaves steeped in boiling water) is a country headache remedy.

Herbalist Nicolas Culpeper wrote in the seventeenth century, "Those that would live in health may use it if they please, if they will not I cannot help it. If they fancy not pottage, they may eat the herb as a sallet."

Watercress in West Virginia is sometimes called a "blood-builder," and the juice applied externally is used for easing rheumatism.

"A lady told me of a case she knew where a man was absolutely crippled till he tried [the cress] remedy, and afterwards quite recovered his power to move and a very good degree his strength," Lady Rosalind Northcote said.

Today we enjoy the wholesomeness and flavor of watercress as a garnish, in soups and sandwiches, and as a vegetable on its own. Here are a few recipes to try.

Cresson Etuvé au Beurre

Blanch cress quickly in salt water, drain dry, and simmer for just a moment in melted butter. Serve immediately as a side dish.

Watercress Sandwiches

Either cover buttered bread with fresh watercress or finely chop watercress and mix with mayonnaise or cream cheese to spread on bread.

Cream of Watercress Soup

Blanch, drain, and chop one pound of fresh watercress. Cook for a moment in melted butter. Set aside. Add four cups of boiling milk to one cup of a white roux made from flour and butter.* Add the watercress, a sprig of thyme, a fragment of bay leaf, and a little grated nutmeg. Simmer for forty-five minutes. Strain. Add one cup hot chicken broth. Just before serving add one cup fresh milk or cream and a tablespoon of chervil leaves.

*White roux is made by cooking flour and clarified butter for five minutes over medium heat, stirring constantly.

Mountain Mint

Our family still enjoys a cup of hot mountain mint tea with honey or sugar in the winter and a chilled glass of iced mountain mint tea with lemon in summer. Just use two teaspoons of fresh mountain mint leaves (of any variety) in boiling water for each cup of tea. Steep for five minutes. Mountain mint leaves and flowers dry beautifully if hung loosely bunched in a warm, dry, and dark place until crisp. The dried leaves are wonderful in potpourri or for tea in winter. Remember to use only one teaspoon of dried leaves per cup of boiling water. A bouquet of fresh mountain mint in the house is not only beautiful, it brings its exquisite fragrance to a whole room.

The plant that still has a few of those fragrant and tiny leaves on Owl Mountain in winter can be nearly five feet tall by midsummer. Country people have called it mountain mint, horse mint, and beebalm, but its botanical name is *Monarda*, only a cousin to the other mints in the huge *Mentha* genus.

Our particular mountain mint is *Monarda fistulosa*, with lovely large lavender flowers from June through September. Just walking through its dense patches sends a wonderfully minty fragrance through the forest for yards around while sweetly scenting our clothing for days.

The lance-shaped leaves grow on square stalks and can be either smooth or softly hairy, giving them a frosty gray-green color in midsummer. The striking flowers perch right at the top with a tuft of long, graceful hairs at the end of the corolla.

Although *Monarda fistulosa* is the most abundant mountain mint at Blackberry Cove, I have occasionally found the smaller *Monarda clinopodia* with its white flowers in clumps on the dry shale near the top of Owl Mountain. You can identify it by the bracts around the flower cluster and the whitish pink corolla with a lower lip sprinkled with pale purple spots. The calyx has very short teeth. *Monarda clinopodia* never grows taller than three feet.

Monarda didyma is the showy red mountain mint that only springs up occasionally in our mountains—usually in the moist and more acidic places near streams. In

New England, though, I have seen breathtakingly scarlet patches stretching for twenty yards. Its rarer relative *Monarda media* has flowers of a deep rose-purple. It is not found very often in the wild, but variations are being sold in nurseries now.

These vividly blossomed mountain mints are sometimes called Oswego tea because they were first recorded by the eighteenth-century botanist John Bartram growing in Oswego Indian territory near Lake Ontario. Settlers made a tasty tea that was particularly popular during the Revolutionary War when China tea was being boycotted by Americans. All of these mountain mints were named after Nicholas Monardes (1493–1588), a Spanish botanist who was fascinated by plants found in the New World. By 1597 when John Gerard published his great *Herbal*, mountain mint, or horse mint, as he called it, had found its way to England. Gerard wrote, "the smell rejoiceth the heart of man" and described how it was used as a strewing herb in "chambers and places of recreation, pleasure and repose where feasts and banquettes are made."

Country people say the broth (tea) is good for curing hiccups, vomiting, and gripping pains of the belly. The freshly crushed leaves applied to temples have been known to cure headaches, and mountain mint leaves steeped in warm honey water were used to relieve children's earaches when slowly dripped into a small ear.

Some mountain folk used it in tea against worms, and I have even heard of it used with salt to cure the bite of a mad dog. Not recommended! Mountain mint was used against kidney stones and gravel, and a granny might have whispered, "Bathed on the secret parts of women before the act, it prevents babies."

Mountain mint leaves crushed and rubbed into the skin are a traditional remedy for soothing bee or wasp stings. One old book on animal husbandry tells us, "Iron or thorne or stub may be drawn out by application of horse mint to a horse's foot." (Gervaise Markham)

But the most magical property of mountain mint is the fragrance from one crushed winter leaf, held to the nose with eyes closed, conjuring up the vision of midsummer in the mountains of West Virginia.

Boneset

Boneset tea is the classic mountain remedy for fevers and upset stomachs of winter flu. Our grandmothers wouldn't be without this gentle herb (*Eupatorium perfoliatum*) that acts slowly and persistently to ease muscular aches and pains, settle stricken stomachs, and bring down intermittent fevers. It was known as being particularly serviceable in the digestion of old people.

Steeping several tablespoons of the dried leaves in a pint of boiling water for ten minutes is the usual method of preparation. This should be sweetened with honey or sugar and taken warm in wineglass full doses every few hours. After four or five doses the patient will often break out in profuse perspiration.

Boneset's name is a little confusing because it was never used to treat broken bones. But an old name for influenza was breakbone fever because of the associated aches and pains, and boneset was the common cure. Other folk-names are ague weed and thoroughwort.

It is a native in our moist meadows, where North American Indians from Canada to Florida first used it and then taught our ancestors its value. Now it is included in the pharmacopoeia. All parts of the plant are active, but only the leaves are gathered just after it flowers between July and October. The herb was hung to dry in bunches in dark, warm outbuildings or pantries. Then the leaves were gently stripped off stems and stored in airtight containers for winter.

The grandmothers were very careful to insist that only plants with leaves that joined around the stem, so that it looked as though the stem grew through them, were real boneset. I think this was because a near relative, white snakeroot or *Eupatorium rugosum*, doesn't have these distinctively joined leaves and is poisonous to both grazing animals and people.

One late morning near the end of summer our grandmothers would take down a deep basket and set off to collect boneset. What a good excuse for a ramble! I find it growing, just as they must have, in the flattened-out clearings of Blackberry Cove, around small streams where the sunlight is filtered.

The numerous flower heads are white and look almost fuzzy. These tubular flowers are clustered at the top of a boneset stem two to four feet tall, individual flowers with a disk but no rays. The large, dark green, lance-shaped leaves are four to eight inches long with the largest at the bottom on the plant. The edges are finely toothed, and the veins are prominent.

Fresh boneset is quite aromatic, but the taste is bitter. Since boneset is a perennial plant, I cut only a few stalks from a patch each year. The grandmothers said it was polite to say "thank you" aloud before the stems were cut. If I find a boneset plant growing alone, I enjoy looking at the white foamy flowers and the distinctive leaves. Then I wish it well and move on.

February

Even when it snows in February at Blackberry Cove, we sense the ephemeral. January snow in the Appalachians squeaks underfoot, and the ice cracks in the gullies at night. But February snow is silent with the hint of moisture as it settles on pewter twigs. Before long rivulets make shiny paths down the silver maple bark, and a pale sun dissolves the fretwork of ice along the edges of our run.

Twenty-eight days long, February is the shortest month and the last remnant of our ancient lunar months. Long ago, before politicians and popes decided to regulate time, country people abided by the natural cycles of thirteen months of twenty-eight days and one extra day. "A year and a day" or "a month and a day" was common in calculating common-law rents and contracts.

Our Celtic ancestors celebrated Imbolc in early February as the time Earth Mother started to yawn and stretch with restlessness. Today it is more often celebrated as Candlemas or the Purification of the Virgin Mary, but for all of us it's the time to light candles, acknowledging that the days lengthen and bring more light.

In early February I look for the fat groundhog who has so many doorways in the shale bank behind our cabin. Isn't she supposed to come up, see her shadow, and sleep for another six weeks of winter? She was up earlier than I on this gray day without shadow, so I still hope spring will be here sooner than usual.

The impatience of cabin fever in February is ancient. Most of us feel that urge to get out there and do something—anything to hurry winter out. Yesterday I worked on the fence and cut branches scratching on the roof. Then I woke up this morning with lazy winter muscles stretched and aching, so I move along slowly to a sun-warmed ledge in the cove, where I find tiny rosettes of lichen and velvet mosses have come alive for even a few hours at midday. Nearby, the tiny wintergreen berries have matured to a spot of red under miniature leaves. Chickweed in protected crevices is the first true green, though. Is it my imagination that the alder catkins have loosened a bit? Do I dare look for a sheath of skunk cabbage pushing through the thinnest glaze of ice?

Before I go to bed on this long February night, I sit by the fire and slowly rub wintergreen liniment into my sore shoulders and leg muscles. The warmth spreads almost immediately while I doze in the rocking chair. Sometime deep in the night I am startled awake by an eerie tremulous wail from the mountain. Our family named it Owl Mountain years ago because at night we often hear the long descending cry of a screech owl.

The fire has long since burned out tonight, but it is the bewitching voice of the little owl herself who has chilled me awake. Henry Thoreau called owls "wise midnight hags" and wrote that they "suggested a vast and undeveloped nature which men have not recognized." Today we call it intuition, those secret feelings from which inspiration flows.

Nearly every culture has associated owls with wisdom, women, and the moon. Ancient Greeks and Romans called her handmaiden of the moon goddesses Athene and Diana, privy to their secrets of the past and future and all the forbidden mysteries of life.

In the Appalachians an owl claw carried in one's pocket would stave off bad luck, and owl eggs eaten in a broth would cure a drunkard. If men or boys looked into an owl's nest, they would be melancholy all their lives, but women and girls could peek into as many nests as they liked. This strange old idea seems to be related to the belief that men should not cross the powers of female magic—still not a good idea!

One December long ago my husband and son were at Blackberry Cove to cut the annual Christmas tree. They had chosen a beautiful symmetrical cedar when Reid looked up and cried, "Daddy, don't cut! There's an owl up there." An exquisite small brown screech owl with tiny ear-tufts looked solemnly down at them with great eyes. They stood enchanted for a few moments and then quietly walked away to find another Yule tree.

The grandmothers in the mountains say when you need a wise answer to a question troubling you, ask the owls. If they call once while you count to nine on your fingers, the answer is yes, but if they call twice while you are counting, the answer is no. If they call three times while you are counting, the question isn't ready for an answer. If the owls don't call at all, the problem is something you can work out wisely yourself. On this night I only hear her once, so my answer is yes, and I slip deeper between cold sheets until dawn of this long night, confident in my hope that spring will come early this year.

February is hope—but it is the last full month of winter, and I know in my bones that sleet and icy winds will keep me by the fire for a few more weeks.

Skunk Cabbage

When the first spikes of skunk cabbage (*Symplocarpus foetidis*) push up in February, the very energy of their life force is generating enough heat to warm the soil or melt the ice and snow around them. Temperatures around the hardy plant have been measured at nearly 30°F higher than the surrounding air.

Although skunk cabbage has the honor of being the first flower of spring, that flower was actually formed underground in autumn. Its strange looking little blossoms are on a dome-shaped spadix, each with four petals, four stamens, and a pistil.

The showy part we notice is actually the magnificent glistening spathe surrounding the insignificant flower. It is dark purple or red with yellowish mottling.

Skunk cabbage earns its name from the strong smell it emits. Some people think it smells like a skunk, and some identify it as a carrion-like odor. The smell is not pervasive and can only be detected close to the flower itself.

Both the wretched scent and the reddish color mimic rotting meat—attracting the first carrion flies of the season as pollinators.

The huge cabbage-like leaves appear as the flowers wither, often reaching three feet in length by midsummer. You can find skunk cabbage in swampy woods or meadows from Quebec to Manitoba and south to Georgia and as far west as Iowa. It also grows wild in East Asia but has never grown in Europe or the British Isles.

Sometimes named "hermit in the bog," skunk cabbage has also been called bearsfoot, bearsweed, collard, cow-collard, Irish cabbage, meadow cabbage, Midas ears, pokeweed, rockweed, skunkweed, stinking cabbage, swamp cabbage, polecat weed, and in the South, parson-in-the-pillory.

In 1723 Thomas More sent plants from Boston to fellow botanist William Sherard in London. They included "a pod with seed enclosed which the natives call skunkroot because of his stinking smell . . . [they] call it smoak because they smoke it when they want tobacco and ere the knowledge of Rum was brought among them by Christians they used to make a fuddling drink of it at their gambols and merry makings."

Despite its unpleasant odor (often exaggerated, in my opinion), the leaves are sometimes eaten as greens. They must be cooked in several changes of water to which a pinch of baking soda has been added. Be careful to distinguish skunk cabbage from the highly poisonous Indian poke (*Veratrum viride*) that grows alongside it and somewhat resembles it.

The rhizome, after a lengthy and complicated process, was used as flour by Native Americans. In fact, skunk cabbage is in the large plant family Arceae and related to the South Pacific staple, taro root.

Skunk cabbage was listed in the pharmacopoeia from 1820 to 1889, where it was recommended for relief from spasms or cramps of any sort—including epilepsy and lockjaw. It was once used as a contraceptive, and folk medicine claimed it caused permanent sterility in both men and women when it was used three times a day for three weeks. A solution from the rhizome was once used to cure venereal diseases, and Native Americans inhaled the crushed leaves to relieve a headache. The raw rhizome made into a salve was said to ease rheumatism, and cough syrup was made from a tiny amount of the root boiled in water.

The dried root with honey was used to treat chest ailments, cure ringworm, draw out thorns, bring on menstrual flow, and expel intestinal worms. Whew! It sounds as though another common name for skunk cabbage should be "pharmacy in the bog"!

Chickweed

The little white star blooming in February is *Stellaria media*, one of the most abundant and most useful of wild herbs. It is a member of the Caryophyllaceae (carnation) family, and it grows everywhere in the world—including the Arctic regions.

The reclining stems form dense mats in cold months and then become more loosely branched when the temperature warms. Flowers with usually five white petals grow in the forks or the end of stems nearly year round. Each petal is so deeply cleft it often appears that there are ten petals, and the petals and stamens do vary occasionally.

One easy way to identify the lovely little chickweed is to look at it with a magnifying glass. A row of tiny hairs travel up the side of the stem to a set of leaves and then cross to the other side until the next pair of leaves and so on.

The more common names an herb can claim, the more useful the plant has been to us, and chickweed is the perfect example. You may hear it called any one of these: satinflower, birdseed, tongue grass, white bird's eye, adder's mouth, winterweed, stitchwort, skirt buttons, chick wittles, starwort, or chickenweed.

Birds have always loved chickweed, picking the prolific seeds from the ground. Small caged birds like canaries are often given entire plants to supplement their diets.

Country wisdom declares if the flowers are fully open it won't rain for at least four hours, but if chickweed blossoms are protected in the embrace of their leaves, watch out for rain. It is true the flowers only open for the midday sun, and while chickweed grows anywhere, it truly loves cool corners. Where chickweed thrives, the earth is rich with minerals.

This little weed has been known since the dawn of time as a broth to prevent or cure scurvy and dissolve thickened mucus in the throat and lungs.

One mountain granny claims chickweed broth is a joint oiler, can dissolve cysts, and pure chickweed juice will remove warts. Chickweed broth also has been used internally by herbalists to relieve bladder infections and externally for pinkeye.

One of the oldest and most repeated medicinal uses is as a poultice. Chickweed has no known toxicity, and it does contain steroidal saponins which make the nutrients highly absorbable.

Chickweed poultices draw out infections, and, according to John Gerard (1597), "in a word, it comforteth, digesteth, defendeth and suppurateth very notabley." You can make a chickweed poultice by simply applying the crushed fresh herb or by simmering the leaves in a solution one-half water and one-half vinegar for five minutes. Cool and apply. Cover with a cotton towel and leave from five minutes to three hours.

Chickweed has been eaten as a delicious strengthening food rich in calcium. In Paris at one time street hawkers actually sold chickweed door to door.

The best thing to remember about cooking with chickweed is to never cook it. It has a clear bright taste when used fresh, with never a hint of bitterness. Make chickweed a healthy addition to any salad or make a special one.

Susun Weed's Fresh Spring Salad

4 cups chickweed
2 cups watercress
1 cup violets
2 tablespoons chopped chives

Mix all together and serve immediately. Try a bacon, chickweed, and tomato sandwich . . . or sprinkle it freshly chopped on scrambled eggs.

Wintergreen

This is the true wintergreen (*Gaultheria procumbens*) with its distinctive odor and taste, growing only a few inches tall on this western slope of our Shenandoah Mountains. The bright red fruit that often matures in late winter or early spring is not a true berry but is formed by the ovary becoming swollen inside the calyx.

The small oval leaves of shiny dark green are usually picked in summer and dried in the shade to make tea or liniment. They contain methyl salicylate, the basis of aspirin. An old-fashioned aromatic tea is made by steeping a teaspoon of dried leaves in a cup of boiling water for ten to fifteen minutes. But the traditional Appalachian use of wintergreen is in a liniment to be rubbed on locally to ease sore muscles, sciatica, or lumbago.

Wintergreen Liniment

Add four ounces of the dried herb picked in summer to one pint olive or almond oil. Let set for fourteen days (can be used in three days if needed sooner). Shake a few times a day. Strain and add a few drops of wintergreen essential oil if you like. Keep all liniments in a dark bottle, out of the sun. Add a tablespoon of glycerin to preserve it, if you are keeping it a long time. Rub the liniment on sore areas several times a day.

The Spiral Gift

And so we come around the spiral of the year. It is not a circle because a circle stays the same as it goes round and round. The spiral circles, but each ring is different.

Summer ends on a different foggy morning or chill evening each September. Deep winter takes its own shape, and spring appears on the spiral with a unique rosy sunrise each Vernal Equinox.

The ancient beat of our own seasons has pulsed in our veins since before the oldest memories, and each year brings a new rhythm.

On some turns, the fallen old willow tree sinks deeper into the soft marsh and no longer sends out its golden catkins. Some of our kind slip away into the dark of winter, their stories and love continuing to nurture us in those shadow-places of our souls.

And on some spirals delicate green shoots push up into sunlight, their roots feeding on the black decayed willow-wood. On some spirals our own lives grow in new directions, and new branches bud on our family tree. They rise up from the Earth herself and are wrought by that great spiral without end that spins round and down into the far past—shaping the very curves of our fingers and the colors of our eyes. They rise up and are nourished in the deep rich layers of stories from our families and friends.

They grow strong or bend, break and sprout anew, in rhythm with those winters of raging storms and springs of clear warm sunshine.

We are not separate from the Earth that births us. The grandmothers sing to us every day that when we feel Her heartbeat and Her rhythms and join Her exquisite dance, we will grow and flourish.

With our cars, our air-conditioning, and our cacophony of electronic voices, it is no longer so easy to feel those rhythms and hear Her lyrics. What was once as natural to us as simply opening our eyes each morning has become cloudy and muted.

The grandmothers know we now must consciously take the time and will to feel the pulse of our own rhythms before we can even begin the dance again.

They know we don't have to give up our computers and our cell phones to hear the old stories. We can slip out of our air-conditioned cars any time we choose—the ancient voices still sing to us. We only have to listen and our hearts will sing too.

This particular spiral of seasons at Blackberry Cove has been a gift to me from all my relations. It is our gift to you.

The Grandmothers' Methods

Several years ago I gave my father a Civil War book for his birthday. It was a reprinted diary of Captain Blue that described his experiences in the very hills around our family's farm.

Although I am not one to read Civil War books, I did thumb through it before I wrapped it in colored paper and tied the bow. The account was interesting because it was firsthand, and I knew the countryside. Then I came across one short passage that held me enthralled.

Captain Blue described how one night a young man in his company was gravely ill. The military doctor came to Captain Blue and said, "I don't think he will last the night. We should notify his family as soon as possible."

Another young soldier overheard this, and when the physician was gone, said to Captain Blue, "I know a granny woman up in the hills. Let me bring her down here to see what she can do."

When she got there, wrote Captain Blue, she took one look at the delirious young man, felt his skin, and left. Soon she returned with a "dark vile-looking mixture from her roots." She sat up all night slowly dribbling that mixture between his parched lips until he could begin to swallow it. Then slowly his fever broke, and he ultimately recovered.

We will never know the name of the granny woman and can only guess which roots she used in her medicine. We can surmise that the young man was severely dehydrated and without the IVs of today would have surely perished. And we can understand how the patience of the granny woman who sat by him all night helped to make him better. That slow trickle of the potion on his lips was as much a part of the grandmothers' old healing ways as the ingredients themselves.

The Appalachian grandmothers' traditional healing with nurturing kindness and using the common plants growing around them is so simple it is almost invisible. It is not the standard treatment by medical professionals or the alternative therapies like acupuncture or high-potency vitamins—although it can include those when necessary.

It is the wholesome nourishing that we rarely recognize or appreciate as healing. It is a mother cooking a healthy dinner every night. It is an aunt making a soothing cup of tea for an angry misunderstood young person. It is sitting up all night with a sick baby. It is knowing the plants and animals just outside the door and knowing that the community includes everyone in the web of life of a particular place.

I believe we still need the grandmothers' old way of healing, and we are fortunate in still having threads of it around us. We just need to recognize it, honor it, and nurture it as well.

The Grandmothers' Steps in Healing

The grandmothers know it is the body itself that ultimately heals, so it is important for us to give it time to work as gently as possible. These steps are really just old-fashioned common sense or folk wisdom, broken down into a clear sequence. Sometimes in the rush of our contemporary world and in the din of pharmaceutical company advertising, we forget the basics.

Of course our latest drugs, techniques, and technologies relieve our suffering and save our very lives. They can, at their best, give us a length and quality of life never before known to humankind. But often we race to them immediately while overlooking the innate wisdom of our bodies as offspring of Mother Earth herself.

These grandmother steps let us see just where herbal teas and remedies fit into the overall picture of healing. They encourage us to combine the ageless grandmother wisdom with the newest medical breakthroughs for the safest healing.

See if each step works before going on to the next step. At times we will go through these steps slowly, such as for chronic but not life-threatening conditions like colds or recurring mild headaches or indigestion. Other times we will zoom directly to the last step for such serious and obvious things as a broken leg or severe, life-threatening conditions. The grandmothers' steps are not rigid, but fluid and flexible like life itself. Sometimes after going through the steps slowly or quickly, it will be wise to circle back, using some steps simultaneously. Trust your intuition.

a The grandmothers' first step is simply to rest, sleep, meditate, or pray. This is an important step. Don't overlook it!

a If the condition continues, the next step is to find out the cause. Collect information. Use gentle hands-on touch. Where does it hurt? Share the story with friends and family who have had similar problems. Read your tea leaves.

a After that, change the energy. Use the imagination (visualization), ritual, color, and laughter.

a If you see little improvement, go on to more focused nourishing and nurturing. Use light herbal teas, love, changes in habits or food, more walks outdoors in the fresh air, and dancing under the moon.

a After trying all the previous steps, begin to use the herbal remedies. Recognize that this is the first step that can create unpleasant side effects. Herbs are wonderful green gifts, but their power can be surprising.

a The next step is to try the use of supplements like vitamins or minerals. Keep in mind that there is always the risk that these can do more harm than good.

a Only in the next step, say the grandmothers, use pharmaceutical drugs or hormones. Know that misuse can cause serious injury.

a When none of the other steps has worked, the last step in the grandmothers' way of healing is what one wise woman calls "break and enter." This is surgery, psychoactive drugs, and invasive diagnostic tests. Know that side effects are inevitable and may include permanent injury or even death. Sometimes, the grandmothers recognize, this step is necessary for survival.

Traditional Methods of Preparing Herbs

Herbal Infusions or Teas: These are easy water-based preparations.

Roots: Use a big handful of cut-up fresh root or half a dozen six-inch-sized pieces of dried root in a pint jar. Fill the jar with boiling water. Put a lid on the jar and let it stand at room temperature for eight hours.

Bark: Prepare the same as for roots. Bark is a misleading word. Herbal bark remedies use the inner bark or cambium layer between the true bark and the wood.

Leaves: Use two handfuls of cut-up dried leaves or three handfuls of whole fresh leaves in a quart jar. Fill the jar to the top with boiling water. Put the lid on and let steep four hours at room temperature.

Flowers: Place two big handfuls of crumbled-up fresh flowers or half as many dried flowers in a quart jar. Fill the jar to the top with boiling water and steep at room temperature for two hours.

The grandmother tradition of healing generally uses simples, that is, one plant at a time, a "simple" mixture.

Dosage: Two cups of an infusion per day is the usual dosage for a person weighing 125–150 pounds. One cup for a person weighing 65–75 pounds. Half a cup for a person weighing 30–40 pounds. A quarter cup for a person weighing 15–20 pounds.

Herbal Decoctions: Simple decoctions are infusions that have been reduced in volume by slow evaporation. Decoctions of roots and bark are most common. Since decoctions are made by evaporation, volatile essences and water-soluble vitamins are lost.

To make: Strain out plant material. Heat liquid until it begins to steam. Turn down heat to very low. Reduce volume to one-half the original. Pour into a clean jar. Let cool. Refrigerate. Some decoctions keep well; others go sour in a few weeks.

Herbal Tinctures: This is a popular way of using herbs medicinally. Small quantities are effective. Tinctures do not retain the nourishing vitamins and minerals of the herb. In the grandmothers' tradition, where the nourishment of the body to heal itself is of first importance, water-based remedies are used first. Tinctures are good for traveling or taking foul-tasting herbs.

Tinctures made from fresh herbs: Gather and chop the plant material coarsely. Do not wash the leaves. Only wash roots, and then let them dry before using. Fill a quart jar to the top with plant material. Fill the jar with moonshine or 100 proof vodka. Cap the jar lightly. Top up the alcohol the next day. Allow the mixture to mingle for six weeks in a dark place. Decant and use.

Tinctures made from dried herbs: Tincturing is rarely suitable for dried herbs. Powdered herbs are never suitable for tincturing. Roots and bark can be tinctured from dried material. Put two ounces of dried root or bark in a pint jar. Add ten ounces of moonshine or 100 proof vodka. Cap well. Watch the alcohol level for a week and top it up as necessary. Decant after six weeks. *Note:* Put tinctures up when the moon is dark or new. Decant them when the moon is full.

Herbal Oils: Essential oils cannot easily be made at home. Infused oils are easy and most often used externally. Infused oils are only made from fresh plant material.

To make: Pick the plant on a dry sunny day. Do not wash. Fill a dry clean jar with the chopped herb. Slowly pour vegetable oil into the jar, poking with a spoon to make sure there are no air pockets. Keep the jar of infusing oil at room temperature for six weeks. Decant. Allow the water from the plant material to settle on the bottom of the jar, and then pour off the oil into another jar. Store in the refrigerator.

Note: Molds grow easily in infused oils if the jars are wet or put in a warm enough place to cause condensation. If your oil molds, discard it and start again. Olive oil becomes moldy or rancid less easily than others.

Herbal Salves or Ointments: These are easily made from infused oils. Pour one ounce of infused oil in a small pan. Grate a tablespoon of beeswax and add it to the pan. Stir over low heat until the beeswax is melted.

Index

Note: *Italic page numbers indicate illustrations*

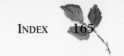